Vagus Nerve Exercises

Activate your Natural Healing Power to Reduce Anxiety, Depression and Stress by Accessing the Secrets of Vagus Nerve Stimulation and Polyvagal Theory

Table of Contents

Introduction 1

Chapter 1: Getting Acquainted with the Vagus Nerve . 2

What is the Vagus Nerve? 2

Where is the Vagus Nerve Located? 7

Functions of the Vagus Nerve 8

The Autonomic Nervous System 13

Chapter 2: How Does it all Relate? 16

Depression, Anxiety, and Stress 16

Trauma 20

Chronic Illness 25

Chapter 3: Activating Your Vagus Nerve 28

Vagus Nerve Stimulation 28

Practical Exercises to Activate the Vagus Nerve 37

Take Care of Your Digestive Tract 38

Shake it Off 39

It's Getting a Bit Chilly Here 40

Diaphragmatic Breathing 41

Meditation, Yoga, and Tai-chi 42

Gargling 42

Exercise 43

Coffee Enemas 43

Massage 44

Passive Methods to Activate the Vagus Nerve 49

Laugh Loud and Laugh Hard 49

Humming and Singing 50
Positive Social Relationships 51
Relax 52
Increased Saliva Production 52
Rinse and Repeat 53
Chapter 4: The Cure of the Vagus Nerve 55
The Key to Your Well-Being 55
From Medicines to Self-Healing 61
Stimulating Effects for All Ages 63
How the Vagus Nerve Affects Your Sleeping Cycle 66
Diaphragmatic Breathing 67
Meditation 67
Relax 68
Using the Vagus Nerve During Pregnancy and Birth 72
Sound Therapy for the Vagus Nerve 77
Chapter 5: Damage to the Vagus Nerve 80
Signs and Symptoms of Vagus Nerve Damage 80
What Can Cause Damage to the Vagus Nerve? 85
Treatment for Damage 92
Chapter 6: What Happens With Overstimulation? ... 95
The Most Common Cause of Fainting 95
Finding the Perfect Balance 99
Interesting Facts About the Vagus Nerve 102
Conclusion 107
References 108

Introduction

Have you been feeling the effects of stress and anxiety bringing you to an all-time low? Perhaps you have seizures or digestive ailments that just don't seem to right themselves?

Your body is a beautiful piece of work, with so many self-healing methods to get you through the toughest of scenarios. In these pages, we will be diving into the human body to have a look at the Vagus Nerve, and the benefits around its stimulation. We will be touching on how you can use different exercises in order to get you through your highest anxieties, as well as tackling depression and severe illness. Learn how to relax an overstimulated Vagus nerve before it becomes damaged, and spot a damaged nerve with ease. Let's get comfortable, prop up with some pillows, and take an in-depth look into what your system can do for you!

Chapter 1: Getting Acquainted with the Vagus Nerve

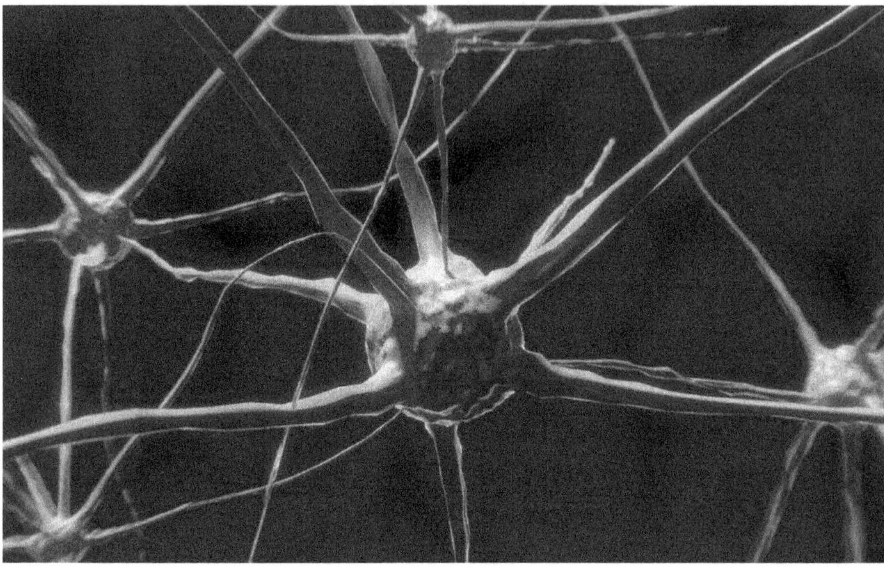

What is the Vagus Nerve?

The Vagus Nerve is one of twelve pairs of cranial nerves in the body. The purpose of each of these pairs is to link the brain to other areas inside the body, more specifically the abdomen, neck, and the head.

Some of these cranial nerve pairs will send off sensory information to the brain and body, such as the intricate details on sights and what you have seen throughout your day, certain smells that may have sparked a memory or left a bad or good impression, a taste that you may know and love or completely despise or that you may remember from way back when in your childhood, or a sound that you find to be familiar for some reason, but maybe you can't quite put your finger on it.

These particular nerves are known to have sensory functions, whereas some of the other cranial nerves within your body will have more control over your movements and well as controlling certain muscles and gland functions. These are better known as motor functions.

The vagus nerve is an anomaly all on its own. This particular nerve has both sensory and motor functions, while most other cranial nerves will only have one or the other of these functions. The vagus nerve itself, you will find, somehow keeps track of way more than we realize.

All cranial nerves are also classified with specific names that are based on Roman numerals. These names vary according to that particular cranial nerves' location within the brain. For example, the vagus nerve is also called 'cranial nerve X' as it is the tenth nerve in the system.

As the vagus nerve is so closely related to many other parts of the body and how they function, it can more often than not be used as a clear indicator of nerve damage when something else in the body begins to shut down or experience problems. Have you ever gone to the doctor and had them test your gag reflex? Say aaah!

This is often done with a cotton swab that they will then tickle the back and sides of your throat with, thus causing you to want to gag. When they do this, they are testing your vagus nerve, and so if you do not have a gag reflex when this not-so-fun part of your check up is happening, it may be an indicator that there is something wrong with your vagus nerve. This would then give the doctors somewhere to start with any treatments needing to be done, when they are looking for the root cause of your ailments. There is not a lot of point in treating symptoms if we can't get to the bottom of everything and fix the problem once and for all.

The vagus nerve is a large factor in the sensitivity of mucous membranes in the respiratory system and plays a massive role in transmitting the strength and rhythm of each breath you take as well as the frequency of your breaths. The vagus nerve also affects the larynx, esophagus, trachea, pharynx, as well as the bronchi, and will also assist with administering nerve fibers to the heart, pancreas, liver and last but not least, the stomach.

The vagus nerve will also have an almost reverse effect too, where not only is it delivering information from the brain to each of these organs, but it is also sending signals from the organs to go back to the brain to react accordingly. In order for this to happen, the vagus nerve contains two separate bunches of nerve cells that are connecting the organs and body to the brain stem.

These cells allow the brain to receive information from the organs relating to their different functions, and can therefore monitor what is happening within our bodies, should the need arise to fix something that has gone faulty.

The vagus nerve's main functions are large contributing factors toward the autonomic nervous system, which mainly consists of two parts, namely the parasympathetic and sympathetic parts. These two parts will be discussed in further detail later in our book under the autonomic nervous system.

So what exactly is it that this vagus nerve will affect, you may ask? Let's have a look:

- Sensory factors such as the throat, lungs, heart, and abdomen are affected.
- Special sensory factors include taste sensations behind your tongue.
- Your motor functions such as movement for the muscles in the neck that are directly responsible for speech as well as the swallowing motion.
- Your parasympathetic functions that are in charge of the entire gastro-intestinal tract, respiratory system, as well as the function of your heart rate.

Other effects from the vagus nerve include the following:

- Delivering information between the digestive system and the brain.
- Deep breathing in order to achieve a higher sense of relaxation, where the vagus nerve will communicate with the diaphragm allowing you to hold a larger breath.

- The vagus nerve will send out anti-inflammatory signals, allowing the body to naturally reduce any inflammation and swelling in the system.
- The vagus nerve can also be used to lower your blood pressure as well as your heart rate, as when the vagus nerve is in an overactive state, it can cause the heart to be unable to pump enough blood through your body which may also lead to organ damage.
- The vagus nerve is also responsible for dealing with stress, fear, and anxiety, which are also directly linked to your gut. This is where the saying "gut feeling" originated. The signals then sent through the vagus nerve will help a person to recover from a stressful or scary situation.

A few other magical moments that this powerful little tool can offer us when used correctly is that it can block the cortisol hormone in your system as well as other oxidizing agents that tend to deteriorate the brain and body and cause our systems to age faster than they should.

We can also confirm that this nerve can help us to overcome sleep disorders so that we may have a more restful night. Great news for any insomniacs out there! This also in turn can help reduce any chronic stress and tension headaches.

Overall this nerve can help us live a healthier, longer life once we have learnt how to use it to our advantage.

Where is the Vagus Nerve Located?

The vagus nerve comes from Latin meaning wandering nerve, which is aptly named due to it being the longest cranial nerve and reaching all the way down to the digestive system from the brain stem.

The sensory components of the vagus nerve are divided into two parts, namely somatic components which help with feeling sensations in your muscles or on your skin, and then visceral components which are sensations that are felt in your body's organs.

Technically, there are two vagus nerves, being the left and the right, but doctors will normally refer to the pair as one whole vagus nerve.

The vagus nerve is in the cranium, much like the spinal cord, and from there it moves down into the neck, passes through a number of organs, and ends up in the abdomen. The vagus nerve goes from the medulla oblongata and passes itself between the inferior cerebellar peduncle where it will then further extend through the jugular foramina and moves in a posterolateral form in between the internal carotid artery and the internal jugular vein along its route down the neck to the chest and abdomen.

This goes to show just how long the vagus nerve truly is, and even then, you find that it goes that extra step further in contributing towards the viscera where the colon lies.

If we split the pair up to have a look at each of the two vagus nerves separately on their way down the nervous system, you will find that the right vagus nerve allows the right recurrent laryngeal nerve to hook itself around the subclavian artery, and then passes up into the neck in between the esophagus and tracheal passage. The right vagus nerve will then cross over into the right subclavian artery itself, and then passes alongside behind the superior vena cava, and further goes down to the back of the right main bronchus. This nerve then contributes to pulmonary, cardiac, and esophageal jungle. It lastly becomes the posterior vagal trunk at the bottom and last end of the esophagus, and from there it will enter the diaphragm.

Next up is the left vagus nerve which then moves into the chest cavity between the left carotid artery and left subclavian artery. The left vagus nerve then allows the left recurrent laryngeal nerve to hook itself around the aortic arch, which ascends between the esophagus and trachea. The left vagus nerve further branches out into making up the jungle in the pulmonary system, then further enters into the abdomen as the anterior vagal trunk in the esophageal hiatus of the diaphragm.

Functions of the Vagus Nerve

One of the greatest anomalies about the vagus nerve is that it is the major parasympathetic nerve of the entire body! This nerve is supplying parasympathetic fibers throughout the nervous system to all the most important organs of the body, especially focusing on those within the abdomen, chest cavity, neck and head. The vagus nerve is in charge of many of the body's main functions that all seem a bit strange to be linked together. Have you noticed that when you clean your ears out and stimulate the ear canal, you cough? That is because the cough reflex is directly linked to ear canal stimulation.

The vagus nerve is also directly linked to your gag reflex when the back and sides of the throat are stimulated, it is linked to slowing your heart rate, and it can control your sweating and regulate your blood pressure. It can also stimulate peristalsis of the gastrointestinal tract as well as being able to control your vascular tone.

The vagus nerve has both sensory as well as motor functions that keep us ticking the way we should. Some of these functions include:

- The stimulation of muscles in the soft palate, which is in the roof of your mouth, as well as stimulating the larynx and pharynx inside your throat.
- Heart stimulation, which thereafter helps to lower your heart rate as well as regulate your blood pressure.
- The stimulation of the digestive tract in order to help you with digestion and passing your food through your system. This also includes stimulation of the esophagus.
- Stimulation of the sensitive skin behind your ears as a sensory piece, as well as sending information to the brain to trigger reflexes when stimulation is

affecting the outer ear canal as well as the throat. You will also find that it plays a part in your taste sensations at the back of your mouth where the root of your tongue is.

When the vagus nerve gets stimulated very suddenly without any warning, you can cause a reaction called the vasovagal reflex to happen. When you get a vasovagal reflex, you often find that it causes a sudden drop in blood pressure as well as your heart rate will slow down dramatically.

There are some people who are unfortunately prone to getting these reflexes although it is most commonly found due to stress, high amounts of pain, getting a sudden fright or even from a gastrointestinal problem from something you may have eaten that didn't quite agree with your insides.

When this vasovagal reflex does happen, it will cause your heart rate and blood pressure to drop very quickly, most often causing loss of consciousness or fainting. This is a condition that is called vasovagal syncope.

When the vagus nerve gets stimulated for therapeutic effects, you will find that you are able to have complete control over your body!

You can stimulate the vagus nerve to stop a nasty hiccup episode that is relentless, and doctors will often use the vagus nerve to help them diagnose a potential heart murmur or to treat depression.

In order for your brain to know the current status of what is happening to the organs around your body, it needs the signals from the vagus nerve to bounce back through those organs and send a sort of 'report' back to the brain in order to react further.

The vagus nerve has become so important in the medical industry that doctors are now finding that they can stimulate the vagus nerve using a device that gets placed in your chest, somewhat like a pacemaker, and send signals to the nerve through this device in order to get certain reactions from your body. Vagus nerve blocking is also fast becoming a popular method of treatment, especially aiding in weight loss as it has become far more superior to that of gastric bypass surgery!

Let's go into some further details on the functions of the vagus nerve in medical cases.

The vagus nerve in relation to the heart is quite possibly the most important case of all. The right vagus nerve leads straight on to supply the sinus node, and can then cause sinus bradycardia when the right vagus nerve gets stimulated. The left vagus nerve leads on to the AV node which can then cut off stimulation to or block the heart when it gets stimulated. In blocking this particular receptor, you are then able to control your heart rate and blood pressure.

Another procedure that has also been made available is called a vagotomy. This is where the vagus nerve gets cut as a form of therapy. This method has been used for decades mostly as a treatment for peptic ulcers, as by doing this procedure, doctors were able to reduce the peptic acid that the stomach was producing. The vagotomy has slowly been weaned away from being a first option in treatment, however, as it was found to have far too many adverse effects on the system in the long term.

Nowadays you are far more likely to find people having treatment on their vagus nerve in the form of an electrical simulator that is placed in the chest, much like a pacemaker. These electronic devices are able to stimulate the vagus nerve if and when needed in order to treat various chronic medical problems. These vagus nerve stimulation devices have been used to successfully treat severe epileptics as well as severe depression when patients were unable to use drug therapy as a means of medical treatment.

The companies that are making these vagus nerve stimulation devices are now looking into the possibilities of their usage for stimulating weight loss, easing fibromyalgia pain, and combating those nasty migraines that you just can't get rid of. This will be a very promising project for the future once there is solid evidence of it working and being a safe method for each of these medical ailments, but in the meantime we can look out for this magic that the future will bring.

The vagus nerve also serves a very interesting purpose when it comes to the flight or fight mode that our bodies go into when something is wrong. Stimulation of the vagus nerve can result in relaxation after a situation that has left us feeling overly stressed or trapped in that fight or flight mode.

It will also indicate to us when we are in potential danger and need to keep our guard up and our wits about us, keeping us safe in the long run like an animal's instincts would. During emotional stress, if the vagus nerve is overstimulated, it can overcompensate for the sympathetic nervous system and ultimately cause a vasovagal syncope as your heart rate can suddenly drop. It is said that vasovagal syncope is more likely to affect women and children than it does men, and can often lead to loss of bladder control in the moments leading up to an extreme fear or stressful situation.

Because the vagus nerve has efferent fibers that pass through the pharynx as well as the back of your throat, it therefore becomes responsible for your gag reflex, as well as having these nerve endings going straight down the esophagus. The stimulation of these receptors can potentially cause vomiting and in the long run, if overstimulated, may also result in a vasovagal response as discussed earlier.

The functions of the vagus nerve in the gut also play an interesting role. These nerves allow a feeling of being satiated once you have eaten a meal. If the vagus nerve is damaged or blocked, the receptors can then cause you to take in far more food than what is needed and it will then end up causing hyperphagia.

The Autonomic Nervous System

The autonomic nervous system is a part of the nervous system that controls bodily functions that are we are not consciously aware of or controlling ourselves. In order for us to understand the autonomic nervous system, we need to know that the nervous system is made up of two opposing systems that are constantly sending information back and forth the brain and back to the organs.

The sympathetic side of the autonomic nervous system is mostly in control of your energy levels, alertness during the course of the day, your blood pressure, breathing, and heart rate.

This part of the system prepares us to act when it is needed and greatly affects hormones that give you your fight or flight reactions, namely adrenaline and cortisol levels. The parasympathetic side of the nervous system which contains most of the vagus nerve's functions and which the vagus nerve is greatly a part of, is there to decrease alertness, help with calming effects on the body, lower your heart rate and blood pressure, as well as aid your body with relaxation in stressful moments and help with digestion. Because the vagus nerve is a large part of the parasympathetic system, it also plays a role in helping with urination and defecation as well as sparking sexual arousal!

You can picture these two systems working together much like the accelerator and brake in a car.

The sympathetic nervous system would be your accelerator and it gets us up and going with all the energy in the world, and then when it comes time to calm down and relax, the parasympathetic nervous system will be your decelerator and will therefore reduce the speed at which we are going, and will then use certain neurotransmitters such as acetylcholine in order to lower your blood pressure and heart rate and cause the organs of the body to slow down their processes, too.

Chapter 2: How Does it all Relate?

Depression, Anxiety, and Stress

When we find ourselves stuck in a stressful situation, we ultimately end up activating our sympathetic nervous systems which gives us our fight or flight mode. If the stressful situation doesn't get sorted quickly and we are stuck in that tense moment, we are then unable to turn off the responses that are triggering that mode. This in turn causes many destructive problems to our systems and can lead up to our bodies shutting down. Our brains then trigger to activate two pathways, namely the hypothalamus pituitary adrenal axis as well as the brain intestine axis.

When we are stressed and suffering with anxiety in certain situations, the brain will respond by increasing the production of your hormone levels within the pituitary gland, where the ACTH hormone gets released into your system through the bloodstream.

This hormone will then travel to your adrenal glands where adrenaline and cortisol will be stimulated. These two hormones will then play a role in being inflammatory precursors as well as immune system suppressors, which explains why we end up feeling sick and worn down when we are stressed and anxious over something. We end up getting incredibly sick easily as our immune systems are down for that time and ultimately we can then slip into a depression which has also been linked to an inflammatory brain response.

We have also found that when you are anxious and chronically stressed, your brain will often have an increase in a neurotransmitter called glutamate, and when it is overstimulated and produces in excess, it can be a leading cause in depression, anxiety, and cause severe migraines.

These stressors that cause a higher level of cortisol in the system can also be a leading factor in memory loss as well as the formation of new memories. When the vagus nerve is involved, or if the vagus nerve gets damaged in any way, it can lead to unwanted symptoms such as difficulty breathing and heart arrhythmia, which often causes fainting spells, dizziness, gastrointestinal problems, and over-emotional responses.

When the vagus nerve has no control over the relaxation signal, the sympathetic nervous system stays active and causes the sufferer to have impulsive responses toward anxiety and depression.

Interestingly, a study that was developed at the University of Miami discovered that when a woman is pregnant, her vagal tone gets transmitted to her unborn baby.

This means that women who go through a stressful pregnancy, or suffer from anxiety, anger, and depression during their pregnancy will transmit those feelings into their unborn child. These women who were in the study were found to have a much lower vagal response to certain stimuli, and their children also had the same or similar response with a lowered vagal tone as well as having lower levels of serotonin and dopamine in their bloodstream.

It has therefore been found that adding vagus nerve stimulation on top of medication for the treatment of depression can ultimately improve a person's quality of life in the long run, especially for those who suffer with severe chronic depression that medication alone may not be helping with.

The National Institute of Mental Health has come to find that over tens of millions of people have gone into a state of major depression during the last year alone in the United States of America, and most of these people have reported that their depression did in fact take a hit on their quality of life overall.

Sometimes the therapies offered for depression just don't quite cut it. Even after making lifestyle changes, being on several medications, and going to counselling, people are finding that they are still not getting any improvement on their quality of life.

Neurostimulation these days is becoming far more popular and fast acting, especially for those with treatment-resistant depression. One of the best forms of neurostimulation is vagus nerve stimulation. In vagus nerve stimulation, a small device is fitted just under the skin of a patient's neck or chest, then the device will send a small electrical stimulation straight into the vagus nerve which will pass its way through the chest, the abdomen, the neck, and through the brain.

A study was done where a team had decided to examine the effects of vagus nerve stimulation on hundreds of people who had treatment-resistant depression. All those who participated in the study had tried at least four antidepressants and had absolutely no success with any of them before trying the vagus nerve stimulation study. Half of the participants were treated with vagus nerve stimulation on top of their current treatments, while the other half just continued their usual medication and psychotherapy treatments with no vagus nerve stimulation.

In order to truly evaluate the participants' overall quality of life, the team used certain parameters in order to get the most accurate results such as:

- The test subject's perceived physical health
- The ability to work, especially under pressure
- The ability to get around, long and short distance
- The test subject's mood at the time of trial
- The test subject's relationships with their family members
- What each test subject enjoyed doing for fun and leisure

The patients who were fitted with vagus nerve stimulators were found to be feeling much better than they had in a long time, with some improving so drastically that they felt little to no depression by the end of the study.

The vagus nerve stimulator has been shown to not only improve a person's ability to focus, but has also been shown to improve alertness and reduce anxiety in the person using it.

When a person feels like they have more focusing ability and they are more alert and active, their stress levels decline and a better quality of life can resume from there. In adding the stimulator to a patient's current medication, it can make a world of difference in that person's everyday life and how they function in society.

Trauma

Post-traumatic stress can have a number of nasty adverse effects on the body including a tight feeling in the chest, a gut feeling where your stomach is sinking, a knot in your throat that prevents you from swallowing, as well as chronic exhaustion that can knock your socks off and cause you to want to rather stay in bed for the rest of the day or longer.

Part of the main healing process that is needed is now directly linked with a healthy body. In such a case, there are now more people turning toward yoga, meditation, massages, acupuncture, and a change in nutrition in order to deal with their post-traumatic stress.

These particular therapies that connect our mind and body in healing allow us to be calmer during a stressful time, as well as allow us not to overreact or get impulsive when chaos strikes.

During these exercises we are increasing our awareness of the world around us and therefore we can make choices that keep us calm and grounded at all times, giving us more control over how we feel in the long run. Many of these types of mind and body therapies involve using and stimulating the vagus nerve.

Our newly found knowledge about the workings of the vagus nerve now help us to understand the in-depth need for its stimulation in order to combat and understand the link between traumatic stress and our ability to heal. In this sense the vagus nerve takes the limelight on treatment with trauma cases.

All of these mind and body therapies involving the vagus nerve are there to ultimately help you find serenity and balance in your lifestyle. We can use a number of breath and movement exercises in order to stimulate the vagus nerve into its parasympathetic state that will relax you in the long run. Through self-awareness and learning about your mind and body, you can find out exactly what makes you tick and use the strategies alongside the vagus nerve in order to restore your sense of safety and to be able to heal from any trauma that you may have been exposed to.

In using the vagus nerve to combat these traumas, we are in the long run able to:

- Improve our mental and physical health
- Enjoy an enhanced emotional lifestyle and well-being
- Have better involvement in society as a whole

- Have reduced blood pressure due to a lack of stress in our daily routine
- Have a reduction in those who rely on and use opiates as well is psychotropics
- Have improved digestive health as stress can lead to an imbalance in gut bacteria
- Improvement of inflammatory problems such as arthritis
- Control and maintain symptoms of Post-Traumatic Stress Disorder

When using a mind and body therapy such as stimulation of the vagus nerve in order to get through trauma, we are then reflecting on our thoughts and behaviors which we can then use to help us increase our tolerance towards distress as well as decrease our emotional reactivity and anxieties. This can also help us decrease pain levels that we are aware of and give us a further sense of self- compassion and show compassion towards others.

When it comes to trauma, we tend to react in a similar way. When our minds and bodies perceive something to be a threat towards us, our breathing and heart rate change.

If we take, for example, how an animal will breathe when a predator is nearby, they may breathe quite rapidly into their upper chest cavity which is showing their fight or flight response using the sympathetic nervous system. This burst of adrenaline that is leased allows the animal a fighting chance to run away in the face of a seriously dangerous situation.

In some cases, an animal might hold itself dead still, and breathe in a very shallow manner in order to avoid being noticed by the nearby predator. By standing or lying dead still, the animal may find that its predator can lose interest in it completely. Some animals will take it one step further and even faint, so that a predator would think that it is a dead carcass and wander past it looking for something fresher to catch. In each of these responses, the vagus nerve is used in either a sympathetic or parasympathetic way.

Once the animal feels safe again, the animal will start shaking and breathing in such a way in order to release the stress response and restore a feeling of homeostasis. We, as humans, however, will generally stay in that high fight or flight activation or the low freeze and faint activation for much longer periods of time before being able to fully recover from the ordeal that we are going through. This is especially the case when our trauma is chronically repeated such as when we have Post Traumatic Stress Disorder.

Secondly, we do not normally have the opportunities required to process a traumatic or stressful moment or event.

When we are reacting to traumas from the past, we are ultimately getting flashbacks of stressful events that then trigger a response to our fight or flight patterns with the vagus nerve. It may be necessary to also work with a therapist in conjunction with getting vagal nerve stimulation, especially if they specialize in trauma treatment so that you can heal from these wounds from the past. The vagus nerve can help you to overcome the fears, but can ultimately only do so much by itself. If the underlying causes of the problems are not targeted specifically, you may find that the imbalances in your vagus nerve will likely continue until the problem has been resolved once and for all.

Symptoms of Post-Traumatic Stress Disorder include a heightened sense of anxiety when put into certain situations, feeling that you may be experiencing the original traumatic event over again in real time, avoiding anything that may remind you of the past trauma, as well as negative feelings and thoughts floating in your head.

Although most traumatic disasters normally come from accidents and physical or even sexual violence, many traumas are also found to come from larger scale worldwide problems such as crime, natural disasters, and terrorist attacks. Unfortunately, there is no way to completely cure Post Traumatic Stress Disorder, and unfortunately current treatments may not always be effective for all patients as each one will react differently to treatment.

Those working in the field of Post-Traumatic Stress Disorder and the pharmacology surrounding it have found that Post Traumatic Stress Disorder is now fast becoming a crisis in the country and have three main concerns around its current treatment.

Firstly, sertraline and paroxetine are the only two known drugs on the market that are FDA approved for the treatment of Post-Traumatic Stress Disorder. These particular medications are able to reduce the severity of the symptoms but will not be able to completely cure the disorder.

The next concern is that Post Traumatic Stress Disorder patients get prescribed a colorful number of medications that are meant to help with alleviating each symptoms such as anxiety, insomnia, sexual dysfunction, chronic pain, and depression, without having the proper testing done with regards to drug interactions.

The high relations between Post Traumatic Stress Disorder and drug addictions are also posing a challenge toward the pharmaceutical industry. The last major concern is how there have been no new developments in the treatment of Post-Traumatic Stress Disorder, and the last medication to be approved for treatment was in 2001 with nothing more recently.

Chronic Illness

The vagus nerve has also been studied and found to show a significant reduction in the symptoms of arthritis as well as other inflammatory issues. The results from a study have shown that through stimulation of the vagus nerve, especially electrically through a vagus nerve stimulator, we are able to find an alternative treatment for certain inflammatory ailments that other treatments

that have been tried and tested may not be effectively working for.
Some treatments are either found to not have any difference in the patient who is undergoing them while other treatments are not tolerated at all.
The results of the study showed that stimulation of the vagus nerve not only helped greatly in the reduction of symptoms relating to arthritis, but it can also help with alleviating other chronic inflammatory diseases.

It is believed that when the inflammatory reflex within our brains gets signaled, the signals get transmitted to the vagus nerve which can then alert an inflammatory molecule called tumor necrosis factor, which is a therapeutic target when dealing with arthritis. It is found that by stimulating the inflammatory reflex in this manor, the correct immune responses can then be activated without causing significant immunosuppression.

In one study, a tiny neurostimulator that was implanted into 14 patients with arthritis was observed to receive a better response from patients with a single daily stimulation than those who were on oral treatment for their inflammation. The groups were divided into three parts, one of which was a placebo group, then the once-daily stimulation group and a four times daily stimulation group.

The results also found that the once daily stimulation group had shown better results than two thirds of the group that was being stimulated four times a day.

The study has shown that the particular device used was well tolerated amongst the test subjects and had significantly helped with their arthritis symptoms.

This support in data has proven itself to be a potential important treatment approach for arthritis specifically as well as other possible chronic inflammatory ailments.

The study also follows a proof of concept which had used an epilepsy stimulator that had been reprogrammed to use on the vagus nerve and it was used to show how it is possible to reduce inflammation as well as improve the quality of life in arthritis patients.

Chapter 3: Activating Your Vagus Nerve

Vagus Nerve Stimulation

Vagus nerve stimulation means either placing a small device that is much like a pacemaker into the neck or chest under the skin. It uses small electrical impulses that will then stimulate the vagus nerve.

Alternatively, there are a number of home-based methods that can also be used to stimulate this nerve. When a device becomes needed, it is usually in order to treat cases of epilepsy and depression that haven't been able to respond to other medical treatments such as pharmaceuticals or psychotherapy.

The device is located under the skin of the chest or neck, with a wire connecting it to the vagus nerve itself. The device can then send signals through the vagus nerve to your brain stem where it can then process the information given to your brain. The device would normally be programmed and controlled by a trained neurologist, but the patient will often receive a hand held magnet too that can also help them to control their own device. There are studies being conducted currently with the hopes that in the future, the stimulation of the vagus nerve can also be used to treat other conditions such as

Alzheimer's disease, migraines and cluster headaches, as well as multiple sclerosis.

We all know the saying, "What happens in Vegas, stays in Vegas."

Well, things tend to work a little differently when we refer to the vagus nerve. What happens in the vagus nerve most certainly doesn't stay in the vagus nerve, no matter how much you try to keep it there. Stimulation of the vagus nerve can affect just about the entire nervous system, as it links the brain to the heart, lungs, and digestive tract.

It also goes a step further and allows interaction with the liver, kidneys, ureter, female fertility organs, neck, spleen and gallbladder, ears, and the back of your tongue. It also helps to release bile and testosterone into the system as well as stimulate the secretion of your saliva and release tears.

The vagus nerve in general is responsible for the reactions given off by all of our main organs, as the fibers of the nerve itself are all connected to these organs. The processing and management of our emotions happens via the vagus nerve between the heart, brain, and digestive system or "gut" which is why we have an intense feeling in the gut when we go through emotional stress. Our emotions are processed between the brain, heart, and gut using the vagus nerve as the transport method for each of these signals.

When the vagus nerve gets damaged or has a problem, there can be many bodily issues that may result such as an abnormally slow heartbeat, weight gain and obesity, gastrointestinal disorders and diseases, trouble swallowing, mild to severe mood disorders, fainting spells, seizures and epilepsy, vitamin deficiencies, and chronic inflammation within the body.

By stimulating the vagus nerve, we have found that we can improve on certain conditions such as the following:

- Heart disease which is a condition involving blood clots to the heart as well as diseased blood vessels and structural problems with the heart itself.

- Tinnitus which causes a buzzing or ringing sound in your ears that you may associate with hearing loss. This ringing noise may be a constant sound or it may come and go.

- Obesity which is a condition of a person's weight, whereby they fall on the larger end of the scale and can develop other secondary issues on top of their weight.

- Alcohol addiction where a person ultimately becomes completely dependent on alcohol in order to function in society.

- Migraines are painful headaches, often causing a loss of balance, eye sensitivity to light, as well as seeing 'spots' or patterns in vision.

- Anxiety disorders whereby a person may experience strong and uncontrollable feelings of worry, stress, or fear to the point that it interferes with the person's daily routine in society and leaves them unable to function properly.

- Alzheimer's disease which is a progressive disease that takes over a person's mental functions and destroys their memory.

- Leaky gut syndrome which is a gastrointestinal digestive condition where toxins and bacteria are able to 'leak' through the intestinal wall, affecting the rest of the body.

- Bad blood circulation which is often caused by a buildup of plaque within the arteries and blood vessels resulting in stiffness in your limbs as well as severe pain.

- Mood disorders which are classified normally as extreme highs or extreme lows. This is an elevation or lowering of someone's mood for a short period of time.

- Cancer, whereby abnormal cells within the body will uncontrollably divide themselves and destroy body tissue and healthy cells along the way.

With vagus nerve stimulation, we can say that approximately 80% of its nerve fibers are meant to send information from the body and organs to the brain, while the other 20% of nerve fibers will send information back from the brain to the rest of the body.

The vagus nerve uses neurotransmitters, specifically acetylcholine, in order to stimulate the parasympathetic nervous system.

So what exactly is a neurotransmitter?

This is a type of chemical that will be released at the end of a nerve, in order to send a message along the nerve from point to point until it reaches each of the organs. For example, if our brain could not communicate to our heart through the release of acetylcholine from the vagus nerve itself, our heart would just stop beating.

Certain substances such as Botox can also wreak havoc with the vagus nerve and interfere with the production of the acetylcholine neurotransmitter. Botox has been ultimately known to completely shut down the vagus nerve, which in turn causes death due to none of the organs being able to function at all. Mercury can also be a nasty substance that causes issues down the line. When mercury finds and attaches itself to the thiol protein in the receptors of the heart, the heart will be unable to receive any electrical impulses from the vagus nerve to tell it to contract.

So in theory, if we have access to certain nootropics such as huperzine or galantamine, they are able to improve the sensitivity of your acetylcholine receptors and can therefore also help to improve the overall function of the vagus nerve as well as promote its health and healing.

There are a number of other factors that can also play a nasty role in vagus nerve damage such as alcoholism, diabetes, upper respiratory viral infections, or if a part of the vagus nerve gets accidentally cut open during an operation. Chronic stress can also lead to inflammation of the vagus nerve, as well as serious anxiety and fatigue that can leave you feeling unsure of what to do with yourself.

Your daily diet can also play a large role in how your vagus nerve functions and is stimulated.

A healthy diet is more likely to leave you feeling energized with your vagus nerve getting all the power it needs to function, whereas a junk food diet that consists of high-fat and high-carbohydrate meals will reduce the nerve's sensitivity overall. Eating overly spicy foods can also cause the vagus nerve to have a moment of miscommunication with the body.

So, since the vagus nerve has control over such a vast amount of our gastrointestinal tract, we can say that when a person has a 'gut feeling', they literally are feeling it in their gut.

It isn't just in their imagination, as these nervous signals that we feel control a vast amount of our lives in order to keep us safe and healthy. These feelings come from the vagus nerve that is telling us that there is a chance that something in the current situation might be wrong.

Your gut feeling is due to a part of the nervous system being stimulated that specifically controls your gastrointestinal tract called the enteric nervous system. This nervous system then communicates with the brain via the vagus nerve.

It has also been found that up to 90% of the main signals and communication that is passing through the vagus nerve is really coming from the enteric nervous system firing away.

Medical professionals have been studying thoroughly the vagus nerve's influence on the human brain, especially in the sense of using electrical stimulation to help combat the effects of epilepsy or depression. Vagus nerve stimulation is now able to help prevent a person from getting seizures by sending mild electrical pulses to the brain on a regular basis, using a small device that is implanted under the skin.

It has also been found, especially with patients who have epilepsy, that this device has another added benefit that goes along with it, which is that these patients felt like their mood had drastically improved after using the device, showing that the benefits of helping those who are depressed can also be achieved.

Vagus nerve stimulation can also be achieved using passive methods such as holding your breath for a short period of time, splashing cold water over your face, coughing suddenly or even squeezing and tensing the stomach muscles in a bearing down motion.

Concentrating on your breathing through meditation is also a gentle and passive way to stimulate your vagus nerve and become more self-aware of all that is around you. You could join a yoga class or meditation class that can specifically teach you these certain breathing exercises.

Alongside the vagus nerve stimulation therapy, you can also get vagus nerve blocking therapy which is similar to using the stimulation device, but will only be used during the day. With vagus nerve blocking, you are blocking certain signals to the brain instead of stimulating them.

For example, you can block the signal that tells your brain that you are hungry and therefore need to eat something. Instead, the vagus nerve bypasses that particular signal and your brain will not get the message that you are hungry, thus reducing food intake during the course of the day. This particular method is often used in obesity cases, allowing the patient to curb any unnecessary cravings.

The vagus nerve has now also been stimulated to help patients who have epilepsy. This form of epilepsy treatment was first performed in 1997, through the vagus nerve stimulator device being placed into a person's chest under the skin and a wire linked to their vagus nerve. When stimulating the vagus nerve electronically for the treatment of epilepsy, the patient may find a few side effects that may become uncomfortable. Should the following side effects be experienced, the patient should visit a doctor immediately to see if there is a way to reduce or stop the symptoms.

- Hoarseness or changes in voice - The patient's voice becomes quite rough and grainy sounding, which can ultimately lead up to our next symptom.
- Sore throat and difficulty with swallowing - The patient may experience pain in their throat that will also affect their speech and daily functioning.
- Coughing - can lead on from the sore throat. The patient may experience a 'tickle' or rough sensation as they speak, which triggers the gag and cough reflexes.

- Shortness of breath - The patient may find that since their vagus nerve stimulator is also directly linked to their diaphragm, they may experience some discomfort in breathing and not be able to get the lung capacity that they may previously have had.

- Slow heart rate - As this little artificial ticker sits in the chest cavity controlling your vagus nerve, it will also control your most important ticker, the heart. The parasympathetic side of the vagus nerve will be stimulated, thus slowing your heart rate as if you had just been in fight or flight mode and it is now time to relax.

- Stomach discomfort or nausea - This comes from that nasty 'gut' feeling we discussed earlier. Your digestive tract reacts to the vagus nerve being stimulated and may end up making you feel quite ill, as if you were going into a situation that you'd rather not be a part of.

If any of these problems continue to occur during your epilepsy treatment, please inform your doctor as soon as possible.

Once epilepsy treatment had been started, tested, and was rolling into becoming a popular form of treatment, it was soon discovered through the epilepsy trials that depression could also be treated using the vagus nerve. When the patients with epilepsy found that their moods were highly enhanced, the FDA approved vagus nerve stimulation as a form of treatment for depression in 2005.

Considering the fact that the vagus nerve has connections to every organ in the body, researchers are now considering that maybe the vagus nerve would be able to help other cases and reduce nasty symptoms along the way.

These studies are now being performed on heart failure patients, those with diabetes, abnormal heart rhythm, Parkinson's disease, as well as severe inflammation from Crohn's disease.

When it comes to such cases as those with arthritis, which affects most of the population at some stage in their lives, studies that were done in 2016 showed that the symptoms of arthritis can be greatly reduced with the stimulation of the vagus nerve. The patients who did not respond to medications for their aches and pains showed great improvement after vagus nerve stimulation, and no adverse side effects were shown as a result of the trials.

Practical Exercises to Activate the Vagus Nerve

Using a vagus nerve stimulating device is not the only way to activate the benefits associated with the vagus nerve. There are many things that you can do from the comfort of your own home that make it just as simple to activate your vagus nerve. These things done at home will be more for your overall well-being and less for your severe cases and chronic illnesses, but you can still benefit just as much. Here are a few of our favorite techniques used to keep everything in check.

Take Care of Your Digestive Tract

The overall health of your digestive tract is incredibly important for your body to function and it also plays an important role in the functioning of your vagus nerve. Your gut is made up of the theocentric nervous system that is a 'microbiome' surviving inside your digestive system.

This little ecosystem contains hundreds and thousands of good bacteria that hold the balance in your digestive system and keep your body healthy and functioning. This good bacteria that lives inside your intestinal tracts allows the body to help move digested food through your stomach.

If there is an imbalance in this good bacteria, or if illness takes over, your digestive system sounds its own alarm of sorts and triggers an inflammatory response within your immune system and therefore causes a wide range of disruptive responses to your body, such as nausea and vomiting as well as anxiety and depression.

You can save yourself the trouble and create a healthy microbiome for your digestive tract by lowering your overall sugar intake as well as finding out about and keeping away from any possible food intolerances and allergies. Doctors as well as nutritionists will be able to help you to identify these problems along the way and will be able to guide you in terms of alternatives to use instead. They will be able to discover the causes of the imbalance in your digestive tract and give you further options on how you can improve your overall lifestyle to prevent any future gut issues.

Shake it Off

We are quite certain that Taylor Swift was onto something here when she sang "Shake it Off"... These words, when associated with the vagus nerve, are inspired by how animals would have a good shake off in the wild in order to release physical tension or to come out of a freeze response after being in complete panic mode.

You can use shaking as a simple practice to release your tension, too! Inspired by animals in the wild, you can use a simple shaking practice to let go of your own physical tension or come out of a freeze response. Firstly, think about where you are tense as well as what has made you tense. Feel through your body to create self-awareness of what is happening around you as well as within you.

Once you have found each spot of tension, pay special attention to each of them and give each spot a good shake out to release that tension. Surrender your body to the shaking and feel the tension slip away from you and out of reach. You may even want to release sounds along with the tension. By all means, go for it! Let it all escape you and once you feel better, take a moment to pause and think about the stillness and calm feeling that you have brought upon yourself.

Feels good, doesn't it?

It's Getting a Bit Chilly Here

So it turns out that exposure to cold temperatures can also give the vagus nerve a bit of a jolt.

This is because exposing the vagus nerve to a sudden drop in temperatures stimulates the cholinergic neurons that cross at certain points. By stimulating these receptors, you are forcing the body to go into a fight or flight shock that jolts you into the sympathetic nervous system. From there, the body is able to calm down using the parasympathetic nervous system, giving both sides of this nerve a good bit of exercise along the way.

If this practice is done in regular intervals, it is believed that your fight and flight responses may lessen over time as your body becomes somewhat resistant to the chaos that overwhelms you.

In order to get this cold shock effect, you can put a cold towel on your face, jump into a cold pool, or if you are feeling very brave, turn off the hot tap while you're trapped in the shower for 30 seconds and allow it to turn completely icy while you stand under the stream willingly.

You could also lie on your stomach and pop an ice cube on the nape of your neck that will quickly cool you down and have your toes curling. If most of these ideas give you heart palpitations just thinking about it, maybe start slow by drinking a glass of ice cold water as fast as you can.

Alternatively, if you live in a toasty warm climate and have sweat dripping off of the end of your nose on a daily basis, you may find this practice to be quite pleasant and refreshing! Whichever way it works for you in the long run, as long as your heart rate kicks it up a notch, it's effective.

Diaphragmatic Breathing

Most people will inhale up to 14 times per minute and in doing so, have superficial breathing. When you become more self-aware of your breathing rate, you are able to lower the amount to a more ideal breathing rate of 6 inhales per minute.

This forces your body to practice deeper breathing techniques and to fill your lungs to capacity with each breath. It's incredibly easy to practice this routine wherever you may be. I'm practicing it right now as I type! This type of breathing exercise especially helps to trigger the vagus nerve and turns on full activation as it is telling the brain that it is now necessary to calm down, even though the nerve itself has not been given that particular instruction directly. In this way, the mechanism is the same as when you close your eyes and tap against your eyelids gently. Your brain will perceive each tap as a spark of light shining through.

When we breathe in deeper breaths, we are making use of the lower part of our chests and moving the diaphragm in such a way that it will promote relaxation.

Meditation, Yoga, and Tai-chi

Meditation is a fantastic practice in order to increase vagal tone.

This is because with meditation you can directly affect the parasympathetic nervous system and allow for positive energy and feelings of relaxation to overcome you. This seems to work a lot better than some other conventional relaxation methods as well as helps to strengthen and stimulate your vagus nerve. You can also use such practices as yoga and tai chi in order to help with stimulating your vagus nerve. These different practices are known to increase your gaba neurotransmitters.

Gaba helps to promote feelings of calmness and serenity in your daily active lifestyle and overall can help to alleviate stress and anxiety. As for tai chi exercises, these can help to stimulate your heart rate and allow you to get the perfect balance which will in turn stimulate the vagal modulation.

Gargling

Another fun way to stimulate the vagus nerve at home is to gargle with water. This action stimulates the muscles in the soft palate within your mouth which are directly being controlled by the vagus nerve.

You can even spice things up and hum while you are gargling to add to the effect that you will have on your vagus nerve to wake it up. Kids also find this particular kind of exercise most amusing and they can equally benefit from it being turned into a family game of sorts to see who can gargle the longest or loudest (letting them win will have an equally amusing effect).

Exercise

Getting sufficient exercise is incredibly important for everyone's overall health and well- being, but what sort of effect does it have on the vagus nerve itself? Exercise increases growth hormone within your brain as well as reversing cognitive decline in the human brain function.

This helps to stimulate the vagus nerve which in turn will also benefit your gut flow, heart rate, and muscles that get stimulated as you exercise.

Coffee Enemas

Here is one for the not-so faint of heart. Did you know that by having an enema done, you are giving your vagus nerve the workout of a lifetime?

It doesn't sound like fun, but your vagus nerve will love you for it! Enemas are somewhat like a marathon or 100 meter dash for your vagus nerve. By expanding your bowel with a coffee enema, you are increasing your vagus nerves activation levels.

This deep (please excuse the pun) cleansing of your insides is accomplished by overall increasing the liver's ability as well as capacity to filter out the toxins in the blood. In the meantime, the liver is also able to cleanse itself of these toxins by releasing bile into the small and large intestines where it is well on its way toward evacuation through your bowels. Your full amount of blood in your body is constantly circulation through your liver at a rapid rate of a full cleanse every three minutes.

If you are retaining your coffee enema for up to 15 minutes or longer, the blood in the system is able to circulate through the liver a few times for cleansing and works much like a dialysis treatment would. The water content of the coffee enema will stimulate the gut into a form of intestinal peristalsis in order to help cleanse and empty the large intestine of any accumulated toxins and bile that have been removed from the system.

Massage

Getting the touchy feelings of a good massage can help work wonders for your vagus nerve, too.

The vagus nerve can be stimulated if you were to massage your feet and your neck along the carotid sinus (or better yet, ask somebody else to do the massaging for you!).

This is located along the carotid arteries on either side of your neck. A good and thorough neck massage can also greatly reduce the chance of a person having seizures, and a good foot massage can lower your heart rate and blood pressure as your body gets overwhelmed with pleasure and endorphins that put you into a completely relaxed mode. You could go for a professional pressure massage too if you'd prefer, where you can have your vagus nerve stimulated with certain pressure points in the body.

Massage can also be used to help babies to gain weight by stimulation of the vagus nerve in order to assist the digestive system.

To use the powers of abdominal massage as a form of a natural anti-inflammatory with the vagus nerve, we will walk you through the steps to this incredible technique, and ultimately help you balance your immune system, calm the body and mind through massage, as well as reduce the production of proinflammatory cytokines.

By having a pressure massage done on your abdomen, it has been shown that you can improve on insulin secretion to help you balance your blood sugar.

By stimulating this part of the vagus nerve, you are also increasing the movements of the digestive tract and its contents.

The combination of manual manipulation and stimulation of the vagus nerve can have powerful anti-inflammatory benefits.

This particular abdominal massage technique that we will show you is easy to do at home in just a few minutes. Ideally, you will want to perform this technique on an empty stomach after eating something a few hours prior. You can start the technique slowly and work your way up as you see how your body responds to the stimulation.

Firstly, you will want to lay down on a bed or on a comfortable floor mat such as a yoga mat or a thin piece of mattress or foam.

Put you hand just below where your breastbone or sternum sits, then make gentle downward stroking movements with your hand down towards your abdomen. Start doing this softly at first with light pressured strokes, then in a bicycle pedaling motion.
Repeat the motion a few times with one hand pedaling over the other.

Once you have repeated the bicycle motion a few times, start to use your fingertips to make small circular motions on your abdomen. You can start this on the top and base of your abdomen and work your way to your sides.
Once you have reached your sides you will need to move your circular motions inward and downward as if you are pressing a meal down from your intestines. Go deeper progressively until you are comfortable with the depth and pace that you use and keep up this firm massage motion for the next few minutes.

Finish your massage with a few minutes of a gentle two knee spinal twist reclined pose that is common in yoga and incredibly useful when it comes to improving digestion as well as opening up your diaphragm and allowing you to breathe a lot deeper. This in turn makes this practice even better for your vagus nerve.

This helps greatly with inducing an anti-inflammatory response, and your body will thank you for it! This is how we start off the pose:

Lay on your back and close your eyes, then exhale as you pull your abdomen down as low as possible and press your lower back gently toward your floor or mattress.

Inhale and exhale slowly and deeply for the next minute while your lower back is opening. You should ideally get about five to six good breaths in during the minute that you are opening up.

Next up, inhale deeply while contracting your abdominal muscles and start pulling your knees up toward your chest. Keep your back on the floor or mattress as much as physically possible during this exercise. (For those of us whose idea of being in shape is 'round', you're probably sitting there thinking "Yeah, right!" but try to give it a whirl if you can. There is no shame if you fall over like a turtle lying on its shell).

Exhale slowly and bring your arms up and out with your palms toward the floor and in line with your shoulders.

Then on your next slow inhale, lift your feet a bit so that your heels are slightly higher than where your knees are, and then lower your legs town the left in a twisting motion (now you don't feel so silly looking like a turtle, do you?) and allow a gentle exhale as your legs go to the floor on your left side (again, try to keep your back and arms flat on the floor during this process).

Do a double check to make sure that your knees are now in line with your hips on the left side, and your legs and feet are stacked on top of one another while your hip has rolled over to the side. Stay in the pose for the next minute while calmly taking your next five to six deep breaths.

Roll your hips back onto your back with your knees above you, then slowly roll to the right side while still planting your back and arms firming on the floor. Hold yourself there for another minute while deep breathing.

Perform this technique for a few minutes every day to strengthen and access your vagus nerve and give in to its true potential.

In doing this, you will notice a marked improvement of reduced stress and anxiety, better food digestion, detoxification of your body, less pain and most importantly decreased inflammation within your body! You will be shocked at the results after a few weeks of just a couple of minutes per day.

Should you have a severe medical condition, though, always speak to your healthcare provider before performing any of these exercises.

These techniques are not designed to cure, treat, or diagnose an illness of any sort, and they most certainly are not a substitute for professional medical advice given. If you do have any questions or concerns with regards to a medical problem, speak to your health provider first and get approval before continuing with our exercises and other forms of health program or diet.

Passive Methods to Activate the Vagus Nerve

Along with all the physical fun and rolling around we have been doing in order to massage our vagus nerves and stimulate them to the point of no return, there are also ways to stimulate the vagus nerve uncontrollably without you even realizing it most of the time!

These are some of the things that we automatically end up doing unconsciously that can stimulate the vagus nerve and help with our overall vagal tone:

Laugh Loud and Laugh Hard

So we all know that one person who has the most hysterical, loud, cackling laugh at the family barbecue, right? Well, that person may just be onto something! It has been said that "laughter is the best medicine," and it turns out that that statement couldn't be more true.

By laughing, your body releases many endorphins into your body that create a natural high. With this, the laughter that you have can also affect your heart rate, your blood pressure, and the way that you breathe, naturally stimulating the vagus nerve and kicking it into gear to start working on high, then gradual dropping back to relaxation.

Laughter also brings about many other movements that we are not consciously aware of doing, such as moving the muscles in our faces, moving our chest, diaphragm, and even your stomach muscles. It's beginning to sound like a good gym workout without the membership card! Find those funny friends and family members and hover with them for a while, or go to see a comedian if you'd like to give your vagus nerve a thorough workout.

Be gentle on yourself though, as laughing a bit too hard has also been known to overstimulate the vagus nerve and can cause sudden fainting, urination, or coughing fits where you end up with the whole family slamming you on the back while you're choking on your own saliva!

This also in turn causes the eyes to tear up. Just another fun part of stimulating your vagus nerve.

Humming and Singing

The vagus nerve is known to pass from the brainstem past the inner ear as well as the vocal cords, so it is only fitting that humming and singing will also stimulate this nerve and give off a calming effect on the system.

In some yoga practices, Bhramari pranayama, or Honeybee Breathe pose or stance, allows an opportunity to use the humming sound to experiment with how the vagus nerve will react.

When you use the Honeybee Breathe position, you need to find a comfortable sitting pose where you feel most relaxed, then cover your ears with your hands and keep your hands in a position with your thumbs facing downwards. Breathe in deeply, then as you exhale you can create a humming noise that will radiate its way through your eardrum and cause vibrations to ring through your ears.

This in turn is also incredible calming and you can repeat the practice for as long as you feel that you need to in order to reach a level of calm that helps you to function.

Positive Social Relationships

Compassion meditation has been shown to result in a more toned vagus nerve. A recent study had people thinking compassionately about their friends and family while in their heads they were silently repeating positive phrases about their loved ones.

This exercise alone showed the power of positive thinking and had improved their emotions such as joy, serenity, and peace by the end of the study.

The positivity brought on by the thoughts of others led to an overall improvement in vagal nerve function and tone, as it was noted in the participants' heart rate differences. The participants were a lot calmer and showed a more toned vagal nerve than what they may have had with simple meditation alone.

Relax

Though this is often a foreign word for those who are addicted to their work and everything surrounding it, it may just be a key part of helping you to tone up your vagus nerve. It is found that most relaxing activities done these days have some effect on the vagus nerve, but sitting and just learning how to chill may be the ultimate trick here. Simply by reading a book, watching children play, listening to your favorite music while being completely lazy and vegging on the couch–whatever it is, take that bit of time to put your feet up and just enjoy a relaxed moment with yourself.

Increased Saliva Production

So this one seems a bit off-putting and you probably shouldn't be engaging in any passionate moments with your significant other just yet if you practice this, but by increasing your saliva production you are also (strangely) tapping into your vagus nerve.

By calming your mind to a point of complete self-awareness, you are able to produce more saliva that will sit in your mouth until your body figures out what to do with it. The calmer the mind, the easier it is to stimulate this saliva production.

When your mouth has now produced these copious amounts of saliva, you will know that your body has gone into parasympathetic nerve mode which will stimulate your vagus nerve that much more due to your tongue being completely submerged and your soft palate affected.

In order to help you stimulate the excess saliva production, you can sit back in a chair, get yourself as comfortable as possible with your eyes closed, take a few long, deep breaths inhaling and exhaling slowly, and allow your mouth to completely relax.

If this hasn't already started allowing the creative juices to flow, allow yourself to picture biting into a sour lemon slice. Allow your tongue to just relax in this little pool that you have created in your mouth.

Now allow your body to relax further and just feel your anxiety slip away. Feel your hands, feet, hips, and legs all relaxing the tension that you may have built up, as well as allow the muscles in your neck and face to become completely relaxed, too. Breathe deeply with this feeling for a little while and hold this position (and your saliva) for as long as possible to reap the full benefit of the vagus nerve stimulation that you have started.

Rinse and Repeat

We aren't talking about your shampoo and conditioner routine with this one, and we don't entirely mean that you need to rinse your saliva production that we just had in the previous step, but we do mean here that you need to repeat some of these vagus nerve stimulating exercises wherever and whenever possible, as the vagus nerve is constantly trying to help us balance our daily lives.

Help this nerve to help you in the long run!

By putting aside a few minutes of your day, even just to take a few conscious deep breaths, you are ultimately finding your balance and toning your vagus nerve. In addition, we need to be able to be safe and in our zones in order for these practices to be successful.

Sometimes after a stressful day at work, when the world is coming down upon you and you think you're about to fly straight into a window like an unfortunate bird, the body goes into panic mode and will tell you that you aren't safe in your current situation.

This is where it is most important to listen to our bodies and take a hint from the vagal nerve that is telling you to slow down and take a minute to breathe and relax. This is how we ultimately protect ourselves and our well-being in the long run.

Chapter 4: The Cure of the Vagus Nerve

The Key to Your Well-Being

So now that we have overcome the feelings and questions of "what on earth are you talking about when you go on about the vagus nerve?", we can now touch on how it generally affects a person's overall well-being, and summarize what we have learnt so far.

When I personally think about health and well-being, I think about a detoxed body and mind, a sense of ultimate calm and relaxation with minimal disturbances within the soul. We have now learnt that with the power of the vagus nerve, we can achieve exactly that! Move over medications and toxins, because a natural method of healing is well on its way here.

The role that the brain plays alongside the body is certainly one of extraordinary measure. We never quite fathom how much our brains can affect our system and overall health but they seem to go hand in hand. By activating the vagus nerve, you are allowing the sympathetic and parasympathetic nervous systems to take over and run the show for you.

Your body almost gets put on auto-mode and instinct takes over to take care of your health and wellbeing simply by allowing nature to take its course.

The role of the brain on body difficulties as well as inflammation found in the body can be quite profound.

If you constantly suffer from digestive complaints, higher than normal blood pressure, mild to severe depression or any other inflammatory condition, we have now given you the key that unlocks the door to your body getting to the original state it was in before all the toxins and chaos of life managed to overwhelm you.

For a long time, the vagus nerve hadn't been a huge consideration in my knowledge on health and wellness.

I had heard of it a few times, especially when going through books on meditation or deep breathing exercises, and it is one of those things that you barely touch on in a Biology class, but you never really go into too much detail on how well the vagus nerve can actually assist you with your self-healing journey. When I thought of self-healing, I wasn't inclined to say "Hey, there's a pretty cool nerve that runs through my entire system and controls what I do and feel!" I was thinking of something more along the lines of detoxing juice diets that are (without us realizing) usually filled to the brim with fruity sugars.

I was thinking of meditation and yoga poses, not even realizing that what we are in fact doing during these meditations is activating the vagus nerve itself and allowing it to do all the work here. I was also thinking of long, strenuous hiking trails that all but knock the gusto right out of us, but we do it anyway because it's healthy right? RIGHT! But this also directly activates the vagus nerve without us even realizing.

Once again, you aren't just putting your body through intense amounts of exercise, you are activating the sympathetic nervous system where your body kicks it into high-gear because it's now going to be a case of, get moving and get home, or potentially stay out in the wilderness to die and be mauled by vultures or other odd, wild critters wherever you may be hiking. Fight or flight mode kicks in and you don't even notice what is truly happening as you stimulate the vagus nerve.

In using the vagus nerve to self-heal, we are becoming so much stronger and finding that even our immune systems take a turn for the better. In stimulating your nerves with a response that makes your body feel that it may be in danger, and then allowing it to fix the problem immediately with no questions asked, your body is teaching itself what is truly a problem and what isn't. In this way, when we get sick with something like influenza, our bodies have figured out a way to go from being under attack to fixing the problem in a short period of time, thus also teaching it to avoid these problems in the future. We will also touch on the effects that medications have on our bodies shortly.

If you were to take off your skin (please don't though) and have a good look at the vagus nerve, you would find that it looks just like a squiggly, stringy nerve that branches out to each of the organs, starting at the brainstem and moving its way down to your gut and colon, much like what I would imagine the back of most of our computers probably look like.

It really isn't the prettiest picture when you think about it, so I would much rather give you a different vision on how the vagus nerve would look if we hadn't just imagined some poor cadaver with no skin. I would picture the vagus nerve as a two-part button that I could now push whenever I needed either a boost or to calm down.

This button would be just under the skin, perhaps in the temples of the forehead, one on either side and if I needed some oomph, I would press one button and if I needed to relax, I would press the other button. You could also picture this nerve as a sort of lengthy singular piano string that you pluck when you need it stimulated. This particular piano string would run all the way down from your brain to your colon and depending on where you pluck the string, the vibrations in that area of the body would vibrate and affect that organ. Certainly a much more 'colorful' way of seeing things.

The vagus nerve can in general be considered the 'mediator' between your mind and body, as it will ultimately be the connection that your brain has to your organs and emotions. This nerve is so well interlinked that it gives you a nasty 'gut feeling' when something is wrong! Way to put a physical sense on an emotional state of mind. When people say things like "trust your gut", what they should really be saying there is trust your vagus nerve. That's what is really hiding behind the curtain at the end of the day.

This nerve just becomes more and more interesting. It is so curious that this one stringy little nerve could potentially run our entire systems. Yes, sure there are other things keeping us alive here and we would never make it without blood and skin and all that good stuff, but if you really think about it, a faulty vagus nerve could just as easily stop your heart from beating or prevent you from breathing.

Our lives are directly attached to this nerve and having it as strong and healthy as physically possible.

"Stimulating the vagus nerve to the heart has a really powerful effect on slowing the heart rate," said Lucy Norcliffe-Kaufmann, associate professor of neurology at NYU-Langone.

This is what essentially relaxes us in the long run, as the vagus nerve connects with the way that we breathe and then will send these messages directly to the brainstem for further processing. The message indicates that we are either in a stressful situation or that we are relaxed.

Put in another way, when we inhale, the sensory nodes found in our lungs will send information up to our brain, and from there the brain will send information back down to the heart to either slow down or speed up accordingly.

Surprisingly, it isn't the inhale that triggers our brain to think that we are either calm or chaotic, but the exhale that specifically triggers the final message to the brain.

Taking deep slow breaths will therefore indicate to the brain and heart that you are calm and that your heart rate and blood pressure can come down as the oxygen requirements for the heart muscle are much lower than if you were stressed and it was beating faster. Should the nerve become severely damaged to the point that it cannot communicate with the heart anymore, your heart will not be able to beat properly at all.

The vagus nerve is essentially the main controller of all things to do with the parasympathetic nervous system.

This system is the reason why we are able to relax and calm down after something exciting or terrifying.

This balance in our bodies plays a large role in our well-being, as the more we are able to activate the parasympathetic nervous system through deep breathing and meditation, the more we are able to lessen the nerve wracking effects of the sympathetic system that causes your panic stations to sound the alarms that then release adrenaline and cortisol due to stress.

Writing this book while at the same time learning further on the vagus nerve has certainly inspired me!

There are so many pathways that we can go down when it comes to using this handy little (or not so little) part of our bodies in order to gain full control over our bodies as well as our minds. Everything is linked together in a neat little package to wrap it all together.

I find myself, as I write this, breathing slower and feeling so much calmer that it surprises me how effective this handy little trick really is. Not necessarily the most fun thing to do when I have work to get done, but certainly effective as I sit and focus on what needs to be said!

If you ever find yourself stuck in a situation where you don't know what to do or say, just take a deep breath in and out and consciously slow your breathing down just for a minute or two. You can put yourself in a calmer state of mind and find the words to use with any situation.

From Medicines to Self-Healing

Medications have an interesting effect on our bodies and minds as well as the way that we function in general. If our intestinal flora and microbiome balance in our gut gets thrown off by the use of potent antibiotics for an infection in our systems, the antibiotics can cause severely aggressive behaviors in those who may have previously been quite calm and passive.

The medications can throw off the entire system. Equally so, certain medications can also enhance our systems, such as how probiotics can keep the overall gut and vagus nerve signals healthy and working in tip top order by keeping the beneficial gut microbe levels higher. This has been shown to also go as far as to prevent Post Traumatic Stress Disorder.

Probiotics are able to help with promoting vagal nerve activity as the vagus nerve has a close relationship to the gut and digestive system . Zinc and selenium are also great supplements for people who suffer from stress, anxiety, and any other mental issues which also ends up linking back to the vagus nerve through the digestive tract.

These days, doctors with their modern medicines tend to baffle me a bit. It's all fine and well that they are able to treat the symptoms of an ailment, usually using one type of medication per each individual organ or type of disease or illness, but at the same time we end up ignoring the fact completely that your vagus nerve and brain are really in charge of the show here and that they tend to tell your organs what to do and when to do it. Your organs will send out a little memo or status check in of sorts to the brain through the use of the vagus nerve to let your brain know how everything is going in there. If there is a problem within, your brain won't take long to know about it and thus is able to act on it with immediate effect.

This is very much a plain and simple part to figure out really. If everything is going well with your organs and vagus nerve, then your brain is happy too. It's a two way street for these organs.

If an organ is struggling and our vagus nerve picks up on it, your brain can be signaled to send in backup and allow for further resources and help for that particular organ. Now if we were to mess with this system by throwing extra medications into the mix, your brain is going to be off balance. You are now going to be feeling better symptomatically, which your brain will also acknowledge, but overall your organ will still be fighting off whatever is attacking it and it will ultimately battle until the brain is signaled by the vagus nerve to lend a hand again.

Stimulating Effects for All Ages

So here is a fun fact that I'd bet you didn't know (until you picked up this book, anyway). You can tone your baby's vagus nerve! Is this not the strangest thing that you have come across all day? We would not be surprised at all if it was.

Needless to say, there are a vast number of factors that play a role in a baby's vagal nerve tone. It all starts from pregnancy! If a mother had depression, anxiety, or stress during her pregnancy, her baby will end up having a low vagal tone.

If anyone has ever told you that an anxious mother creates an anxious baby, this is exactly why that statement is true. Babies that are born prematurely, before they were meant to be born, will also be found to have a low vagal tone. These are the babies that it would be best suited to give a few vagus nerve exercises to and help them to stimulate their vagus nerve better, allowing it to become stronger and healthier as they grow into the little terrors that we know and love.

If you found that you went through a rough pregnancy and your world just fell apart around you for a chunk of your three trimesters, don't worry at all, it really isn't the end of the world for you or your infant. You are able to easily help to tone your baby's vagus nerve simply by going through your usual bonding time and giving your little one love and care.

Holding your baby against your chest in the classic skin to skin pose is a great way to help your baby with vagus nerve stimulation. This bonding technique will allow your baby to instantly calm down as he or she listens to the soft thrumming sound of your heartbeat. You could also use infant massage to get things moving with your baby's vagus nerve.

While your baby is an infant you should probably be nice and gentle with your youngster, especially when he or she can't quite defend themselves against an icy spray of cold shower water that may not go down to well in the book of forgiveness later on.

You can, however, use a cool wet wipe to wipe your baby's face and blow cool air on them, or if it's cool outside versus your indoor temperature you could have a short walk in your garden to give your little one a mild cold shock. Just try not to make them sick while doing so.

Once your baby has aged enough to agree to a cold shower, you can then look at some more adult friendly ways to stimulate the vagus nerve that your child is more likely to understand such as breathing techniques to calm down (this will be incredibly helpful in those first couple years of extreme tantrums and thinking that the world revolves around them!).

A gentle child-friendly massage, or a moms and tots yoga class, along with a few minutes of goosebumps and gleeful squeals in the shower are definitely worth the benefits that your child is able to get out of stimulating the vagus nerve.

By allowing your child to exercise these parts of the body and doing these practices on a daily basis, you are toning the vagus nerve to extend throughout your youngster's body and to go through every major organ in the body and back. A healthy, happy child will lead to a healthy, happy, (sane) parent.

When the vagus nerve stimulating device was undergoing trials for epilepsy, there were children amongst the patients that were being tested. These children were all over the age of 12 years old and all under 16 years old. Most of these controlled studies were done on adults, but with the epilepsy study it was found that the vagus nerve stimulator device has more efficacy as well as overall safety for these children than that of antiepileptic drugs. It is now up to the FDA to figure out the answers to when a child is considered to have severe enough epilepsy for a stimulator to be fitted.

Overall, we can say that electronic vagus nerve stimulation has been used and tested in both adults and children with good to varying success rates. Based on the trials done so far, it would appear that using vagus nerve stimulation on very young children with epilepsy that is potentially life-threatening can be incredibly effective in improving that child's overall quality of life. Larger groups with further studies will allow us to further research and verify all findings thus far.

How the Vagus Nerve Affects Your Sleeping Cycle

When it comes to sleep, you can normally find one of two types of people; those who seem to barely put their heads on their pillows and they are lights out, gone, a bomb could go off next to them and they wouldn't budge.

Then you get those who battle sleep and have a terrible habit of wandering around from room to room aimlessly, trying to find things to entertain themselves at 2am because sleep just isn't on the table right now (I know a few of these personally).

Now, however, we have learnt that we can use the vagus nerve along with vagus nerve stimulation in order to help us sleep better at night and make the most of the hours we need to rest.

By doing a few very simple exercises to stimulate your parasympathetic nervous system before you close your eyes and drift off to dreamland, you can control how well you sleep through the night, down to making sure that you get sufficient REM sleep time, as well as ensuring that you are more alert during your waking and working hours.

If you were to follow some of the breathing and meditation steps mentioned earlier, you may just find a new cure for your insomnia! This may sound a bit repetitive, but bear with me as I can't say this enough. These tips are going to give you a whole new lease on life! Let us go over a few key tips again and see just how they can help with your sleeping cycle.

Diaphragmatic Breathing

This type of breathing exercise especially helps to trigger the vagus nerve and turns on full activation as it is telling the brain that it is now necessary to calm down, even though the nerve itself has not been given that particular instruction directly.

When we breathe in deeper breaths, we are making use of the lower part of our chests and moving the diaphragm in such a way that it will promote relaxation. This is especially helpful when it's bedtime. You could lie in bed quite calmly with your eyes closed and focus all your energy into your breathing. Make sure to take a deep inhale and slowly exhale, allowing approximately six breaths per minute if not fewer. This slows your heart rate right down and will allow your brain to start switching off for bed.

Meditation

With meditation, you can directly affect the parasympathetic nervous system and allow for positive energy and feelings of relaxation to overcome you. This practice is known to increase your gaba neurotransmitters.

Gaba helps to promote feelings of calmness and serenity in your daily active lifestyle and overall can help to alleviate stress and anxiety. Gaba can also be taken in nootropic form, but is far better when you are able to stimulate it yourself naturally through the vagus nerve. When you meditate you are allowing your entire body to become completely self-aware and you go into a state of intense calmness.

This is the ultimate time to allow yourself to drift into dreamland, as it will allow for maximum REM sleep throughout the night.

Relax

I know it can be difficult to just *relax* whenever the feeling strikes, but when it is time to sleep, this is a key part of getting your mind into the zone. You need to become aware of each and every muscle that is tense within your body and physically relax that particular muscle as you go before bed.

My favorite thing to do every night, and I have been doing this for many years now in order to help me sleep like an absolute baby, is to lie in my bed and close my eyes, then in my mind I picture a warm glowing light slowly circling my body from limb to limb. That sounds strange, but give it a try tonight and see just how relaxing it truly is.

Use your imagination with me for a moment. Picture yourself floating. Nothing in the space around you, nothing can harm you, nothing can touch you. You're just floating there in darkness with your eyes closed and you can see nothing. Now start at your feet and picture a warm white light revolving around your foot, starting at your toes and with every revolution that this warm, white light makes, you become acutely aware of the muscles in your foot relaxing and releasing any tension that may have gathered through the day.

Then this warmth continues to ascend up your leg to your calf, still slowly circling around you but not touching you, and you feel the tension leaving the muscles in your leg to the point that it feels light as a feather.

Repeat this circle of light for your other leg individually and continue moving all the way up each body part, feeling your hips completely relax and your abdominal muscles release.

Feel your spine getting the warm light radiating through you as it revolves around your torso; allow each beam to separate again going around each hand and all the while you become completely aware of the tension in your fingers all the way up to your arms leaving your body and your body becoming lighter. This goes for each muscle in the face, too, as you may find that you hold a lot of tension in your facial muscles.

Feel your tongue go lax in your mouth, your jaw become completely loose and able to drop, your neck and shoulders release all tension, and even (oddly enough) the muscles in your forehead relax as the warm light revolves around your head. Are you still awake in there? Just checking.

If this relaxation technique doesn't at least partially knock you out, then we need to re-evaluate the severity of your sleeping problems!

This entire meditation/ relaxation process should take all of 10 minutes, and I even find that I pass out cold before I'm finished with the entire routine most nights! It is the ultimate relaxation mode that, along with slow, deep breathing, can tone your parasympathetic nervous system brilliantly.

When it comes to using a vagus nerve stimulator that has been implanted into the chest or neck, it has been studied that the effects of sleepiness during the day were greatly improved, giving the patient far more energy during the daytime as well as allowing far more restful evenings where the patient did not toss and turn, or wake up throughout the night.

Using a sleep diary, a patient in a study described an improvement of daytime sleepiness with chronic use of the vagus nerve stimulator. The patient did also find, however, that there was a marked increase in snoring after implantation of the vagus nerve stimulator, which was corrected quite easily, simply by lowering the pace at which the stimulator set off an electrical charge to the patient's vagus nerve.

Another study had also reported that an adolescent patient who was being treated for epilepsy using a vagus nerve stimulator showed an improvement in the perception of well-being as well as finding an improvement in cognition, school performance, language skills, and a decrease in irritability. Quality of life was also evaluated in all patients that had been studied during these sleep cycles, and findings showed a marked improvement related to decreased sleep latency.

Sleep apnea has also been seen as a big problem that can be controlled through the vagus nerve. Objective evaluation using polysomnography technology has shown a relationship between sleep disturbances in some patients and vagus nerve stimulation.

During the vagus nerve stimulators period of being on and working, in all cases, the occurrence of mild to moderate sleep apnea was directly linked with the vagus nerve stimulator, and turning it off, or adjusting the setting with decreased stimulation parameters, achieved a control over the respiratory system in most patients. Others required positive pressure ventilation.

Two further studies described the presence of vocal cord adduction during the vagus nerve stimulators on stimulation period, evidenced by indirect laryngoscopy, and then further associated with the sudden onset or worsening of respiratory sleep disorder which is then suggesting a possible explanation for the mechanism by which the stimulator, on a higher frequency, induces sleep apnea.

Using the Vagus Nerve During Pregnancy and Birth

So here is an odd one that you never thought you'd see. Women can use the power of the vagus nerve to their advantage during pregnancy as well as on the birthing table itself!

Pregnant women are notoriously known for completely stressing out at all times (it's not overreacting, it's just freaking out a bit and it is completely normal okay!) because their hormones are all over the place and there's so much to do and this person has been stressing them out but their husband didn't do something along the way and their mother in law is on their back while the kids just aren't listening to anything that is being said and they, themselves, are just about trying to kill each other because someone stole the other one's toy and just *aaaah!* Right Mama Bear, just calm down and breathe.

There really is just no winning for these poor women of our society. So what can they do to actually get somewhere along the way?

Why, they can use gentle vagus nerve stimulation to calm themselves down, of course! (What else do you think we were possibly going to suggest at this point?).

When these darling carriers of the next generation are troubled, their sympathetic nervous systems are kicking into high gear and they end up doing some extra harm that they might not even realize.

In going through a severely stressed pregnancy, or potentially having a moment of depression or anxiety if things aren't quite going their way, their vagal tone as well as that of their unborn baby decreases.

A mother's unborn child will pick up on their mother's emotions and feelings and often arrive to the new world with similar emotions and feelings. This is why it is often said that an anxious pregnancy will lead to a 'niggly' baby. Teenage years don't seem to make things any easier later on in life either, so a mother's work is never done.

This doesn't have to be the case, though! A mother does have options here. They just so happen to be less spoken of while sitting in the doctor's rooms waiting for the next scan.

An expectant mother can use (almost) any and all of the above mentioned techniques to calm herself down when things get out of hand. When I say almost, I mean that I wouldn't recommend the turtle back type yoga that will leave her stuck on the floor with no other way to get up. That itself will be a touch of added stress right there, along with the pains and aches of the round ligament that will be pulling while this poor woman struggles her way back to her feet. Breathing exercises and meditation, however, while surrounded by comfortable supportive pillows of course, can greatly reduce the stress put on an expecting mother as well as her baby.

We are then tapping out from the sympathetic nervous system and tapping into the parasympathetic nervous system in order to strengthen the mother's vagal tone as well as that of her baby.

No matter what the situation is, a mother can breathe her way through all the stress of life. This is at least until it's go-time and breathing exercises go flying out of the window.

Or do they?

Some birthing classes will teach expecting parents exactly how to breathe their way through a birth. For a mother, this means breathing her way through each contraction and focusing all of her energy on pushing this watermelon of a head through her, well, yes. That. For an expectant dad, he could also make use of most of these breathing exercises, as he is going to need to get through having the little bones of his hand severely crushed under the sheer force of his woman's wrath.

Enough joking around about pain, though.

A woman can also tap into her parasympathetic nervous system when it comes time to push. Some women have even said that they were able to 'breathe the baby out'. This was quite a fascinating idea for me, so I took things a step further and went to a number of different mothers to awkwardly question them on their birthing experiences, as well as speaking to a number of midwives and doulas who were also able to shed some light on the subject.

It turns out that if a mother is able to master the art of concentrating on her breathing and breathe slowly, there is a good chance that she may have a safer, easier birthing experience that may not involve masses of tearing and screaming.

Yes, there will most probably be a point in time where she may be quite happy to pack her bags and call it quits at the hospital, ready to walk right out of there, but with the right breathing techniques under their belt, mothers can be powerful warriors during this process.

A woman who is birthing is essentially able to focus on her baby alone and zone the rest of the world out. The contractions that she experiences are also helped along by the vagus nerve, so that every time she contracts, a message is sent through to the brain telling her to bear down and push to allow her baby to move through the birth canal.

Every time one of these contractions happens, the stomach muscles are also helping out by squeezing around the rear side of the baby and also moving him or her in the right direction. By having a mother gently breathe through these contractions instead of giving it all the force she has in her, she is consciously allowing her cervix to relax which is a vital part of birthing without tearing. Her pelvic bones will also be able to move more freely as her baby passes through her.

When a woman is getting an induction or other medications that speed this process along, it messes with the vagus nerve so that the nerve battles to communicate with the brain as to how the progression of birth is going. This sends the vagus nerve into panic mode and whether the mother wants to or not, will automatically tap into her sympathetic nervous system leaving her panicking in fight or flight mode.

This then also stresses out her baby and will often lead to an emergency C section due to the birth canal contracting and not allowing for any progress, as well as the pelvis itself tensing up and not allowing for a natural birth without stressing the unborn baby further.

These medications can also cause some vagus nerve damage in the long run, where it may not function well after birth and will need healing itself.

Symptoms of this damage after giving birth include but are not limited to mild to severe back pain in the spine and tailbone, abdominal pains due to the digestive system being thrown off by the damage as well as having the muscles of her abdomen forced to move in ways that they were never ready to move in, and headaches from the drops and spikes in blood pressure.

Other symptoms include stress becoming less and less controllable for the mother, sore throat and ears due to these parts of the body being so close to the brainstem and beginning of the vagus nerve (not including the fact that the mother is going to be straining, groaning, and grunting through the entire birthing process like a wild animal), irregular heartbeat due to the vagus nerve no longer being in control of, or having the ability to calm the mother down using feel-good endorphins like oxytocin to calm everything down, as well as a sudden drop in blood pressure, which can also be incredibly dangerous for both mother and baby due to it being a common cause of fainting or unconsciousness, often resulting in the mother being rushed into an emergency cesarean section as she is no longer able to push in that moment. If any symptoms are coming up that may be of concern, check in with your ob gyn or family health practitioner to make sure that everything is still on track with you and your soon-to-be bundle of joy and just make sure that your birth plan is still possible and rolling before you get in there at go-time and everything flies out the window, causing even more unnecessary stress on you and your baby.

Sound Therapy for the Vagus Nerve

Your hearing and the ears themselves have an intense relationship to the rest of the body due to their close proximity to the vagus nerve.

The vagus nerve does not play an active part in the process of hearing, therefore it is not normally taken into a lot of consideration in things that relate to listening, music, and anything else outside of the medical field. However, this exceptionally intricate nerve is connected with the rear wall of the auditory canal, the lower part of the eardrum's membrane and in the middle ear.

Because everything is ultimately connected through the vagus nerve, we could say that stimulating the ear means stimulating all the vital vegetative internal organs. This therefore makes the ear and all the things that you hear a large part of the parasympathetic nervous system as it uses that innervation of the vagus nerve to affect the whole body.

The vibrations of sound resonating through your ears will tend to have an impact on all the areas of the body reached by this important nerve by resonating very close to it in the eardrums. In addition, the majority of all cranial nerves are either directly or indirectly connected with the ear.

This is one of the many reasons why the use of sound therapy instruments, such as Tibetan singing bowls as well as tuning forks, can be so instantly calming and relaxing. These are often used during massage and relaxation therapies to chime in the background for spiritual self-awareness, thus also helping the body to come back to the original state that is the opposite of the "fight or flight" mode triggered by stress.

The sounds that you hear will instantly calm you down and allow you to release that cortisol and adrenaline that you may have felt previously. In fact, long and sustained sounds tend to be soothing and relaxing whereas sharp and abrupt sounds tend to trigger alertness, panic, and alarm.

A simple practice of singing, humming, or using your vocal cords in any way can have some tangible calming effects by virtue of its auditory stimulation of the vagus nerve.

You can have a similar effect to what a vagus nerve stimulator can do for you simply by using the sounds of your voice as well as vibrations in order to self-soothe.

When a baby is being developed in their mother's uterus, the auditory system and its nerves become completely functional. The acoustic nerve is said to start myelinise during the sixth month of a woman's pregnancy, whereas the neocortex only completes myelination around the adolescence stage of the child. Myelin is an essential component within the nervous system.

It is a coating substance that isolates the nerves and enhances the transmission of electrical signals.

Before birth, even the area in the temporal lobe of the brain where sound signals are received becomes functional, and the inner ear reaches its full adult size. This is all due to the fact that while we are still hanging out in our mother's uterus, we can't rely on our sense of sight as there really isn't much to see there even if we wanted to. We can, however, start receiving vitalizing signals from the environment via the ideal medium of water in which sound travels very effectively.

This is why it is always a great idea to pop on some of your favorite feel-good music and have a little dance party around the house while going on about your day during a pregnancy. Your mood will be uplifted as well as that of your child without you even realizing it.

It truly is incredible how our brains are wired in such a way that we can put so much importance on sound! The next time you are trying to relax or activate your parasympathetic nervous system, take a moment to listen to some relaxing music or sing along to your favorite jams. It will tone and help your vagus nerve greatly while putting you in a mood that you will never want to escape from.

Chapter 5: Damage to the Vagus Nerve

Signs and Symptoms of Vagus Nerve Damage

Damage to the vagus nerve can have a wide range of symptoms, as this particular nerve is so long and affects many areas of the body. These damages can often range from something mild and well-controllable to that of a full blown problem that requires a bit more attention in order to be solved. You can look out for the following symptoms that may show potential vagus nerve damage:

- Difficulty speaking or loss of voice - When your voice box just doesn't want to play along, it can get quite difficult to communicate with anyone let alone figure out what is happening to you. The voice box is closely related to the vagus nerve and is in very close proximity, so when this nerve gets damaged along the way, you can be sure that talking about it could get pretty tough.
- A voice that is hoarse or wheezy - Your throat is absolutely going to be scratchy and sore. You may even find that your lungs are feeling a bit "iffy"

too, and that will cause you to wheeze and battle when you're trying to speak to someone.

- Trouble drinking liquids - Your swallowing reflex is going to be affected too, as the esophagus is also going to be a fun part that won't want to play along.
- Loss of the gag reflex - If your gag reflex has gone out the window, it could very well be a sign that your vagus nerve isn't playing along either. A doctor will often use a swab of sorts to tickle the back and sides of your throat in order to test your gag reflex, and if you aren't almost choking on the swab by the time he or she is done with you, then you can almost be certain that the vagus nerve has something to do with it.
- Pain in the ears - The ears are very closely related to your vagus nerve as we saw in the previous chapter. If you are experiencing pain in an ear, it could just be from a minor infection, although it could also very well be from the vagus nerve wreaking havoc with your system. If you see a healthcare provider for your ear ache, they will be able to shine a light into the ear canal in order to check if there is anything wrong with the inner, middle, or outer ear itself, or whether it could be that your vagus nerve is damaged and is the cause for the pain.
- Unusual heart rate - If your heart is currently either going way too fast without having run a marathon in the Olympics, or even if it seems to

be unreasonably slow, it may indicate that the vagus nerve has been affected and is causing either the sympathetic or parasympathetic nervous system to work overtime. This is a very serious symptom and should be dealt with immediately by a doctor or healthcare practitioner. Delaying the process of seeking help can potentially be fatal, so get it sorted sooner rather than later.

- Abnormal blood pressure - This is also very closely related to the unusual heart rate. If your blood pressure suddenly spikes or drops without warning, you can ultimately send dangerous signals to your brain in order to get moving and start solving the problem. If the vagus nerve is damaged, the chances of those warning signals reaching the brain are slim to none and can cause severe damage in the long run.

- Decreased production of stomach acid - Naturally, if the vagus nerve isn't in optimal condition, neither is your digestive system. This means that you will also have decreased production of stomach acid, leading to a rather painful system when it comes down to bowel movements. This will also prevent your body from soaking in any vital nutrients through the intestines and stomach lining and what goes in, will most likely come out in the exact same fashion.

- Nausea or vomiting- Nausea and vomiting are also closely related to how the stomach reacts when the vagus nerve is under stress or damaged in any way. If there is damage to the vagus nerve, the body sees this as an illness and will most of the time try to purge out what may be causing the problem. Thus, even though the problem itself is nothing that you may have eaten or ingested, your stomach may still react by releasing bile into the intestines causing mild to severe nausea and vomiting.

- Abdominal bloating or pain - when the vagus nerve is under attack, you may experience excessive abdominal pain or possibly bloating due to the nerves that are directly connected to the intestines and digestive system.

The symptoms that a person might have depend on what part of the nerve is damaged.

It is also believed through some research that damage to the vagus nerve could possibly cause a condition called gastroparesis. This condition will directly affect the involuntary contractions of the digestive system, thus preventing your stomach from emptying itself properly of any digested food.

Gastroparesis will usually show a number of symptoms including:

- Nausea or vomiting, as there may sometimes be undigested food sitting inside the stomach for a few hours after eating.
- A feeling of fullness or overall loss of appetite shortly after starting to eat a meal, as your stomach muscles are contracting and becoming

smaller and not able to add in extra food along the way.

- Acid reflux can often become problematic as with the contracting muscles, your stomach muscles are pushing up digestive enzymes into your intestines and up the esophagus which burns its way through your system.
- Abdominal pain or bloating is caused by the painful contractions of the stomach muscles. Almost similar to that of a pregnant woman in the early stages of labor, things can get fairly uncomfortable quickly.
- Fluctuations in blood sugar which can often be caused by insulin spikes in your bloodstream due to undigested food that sits in your gut.
- Unexplained weight loss

Gastroparesis can also sometimes be caused by a person undergoing a procedure called a vagotomy where a piece of the vagus nerve gets severed for medical purposes, such as for weight loss instead of using gastric bypass surgery.

Sometimes the vagus nerve overreacts to certain stress triggers which is called vasovagal syncope. Some of these stress triggers can be the following:

- Fear of bodily harm
- Extreme temperature changes such as intense heat and cold

- A fear of needles along with having blood taken or the sight of blood
- Battling to have a bowel movement or straining in the bathroom in general
- Long periods of standing without rest

What Can Cause Damage to the Vagus Nerve?

Vagotomy is a term used for when the vagus nerve is surgically cut during a procedure in order to achieve a desired result. This is a now-obsolete therapy that used to be used in order to treat peptic ulcer disease. Getting a vagotomy done is, at the moment, seen as a possibly less invasive way to have weight loss surgery, as an alternative to gastric bypass surgery. When this particular procedure is done, the nerve is cut in a particular place in order to curb feelings of hunger as well as those pesky cravings of sugary junk food. Imagine for some reason deciding that you don't actually feel a need to demolish that tub of ice cream that is sitting in your freezer. Would you do it if you had the option? This procedure will also sometimes go hand in hand with having a gastric band put over your stomach just to make certain that there is no chance that you will be overeating unnecessarily. This combo can help reduce excess weight by up to 43% over a period of six months! Certainly better than I have ever done with my poor attempts at yo-yo diets.

Having a vagotomy can potentially cause a number of serious side effects. This includes such effects as having a vitamin B12 deficiency after a few years of life without that piece of vagus nerve, which tends to turn out to have similar symptoms to pernicious anemia. The vagus nerve is also very well known for its ability to stimulate the parietal cells in the stomach and intestines, in order to secrete acid. The vagus nerve is also known for stimulating the stomach parietal cells in order to secrete intrinsic factor, which is needed in order to absorb vitamin B12 from food into your body's system. When you get a vagotomy done, you are directly reducing this secretion and ultimately leading yourself straight toward this vitamin B12 deficiency which, if left untreated, can cause mild to severe nerve damage to other nerves in the body, increased tiredness or exhaustion during the day, dementia, paranoia, and at the end of all the chaos can result in death.

Researchers from the Aarhus University and the Aarhus University Hospital have also demonstrated that when a person gets a vagotomy done, they are at risk of potentially developing other major diseases later in life such as Parkinson's disease. This is also because Parkinson's disease begins within the gut, in the gastrointestinal tract, and from there will spread itself up to the brain through the use of the vagus nerve. By severing that tie between the digestive tract and the brain, you are able to prevent Parkinson's disease from taking over a person's mind. We can also take a deeper look into the theory that dysregulated environmental stimuli, which is often received and passed along between the digestive system and the vagus nerve, may also have a nasty effect on the dopamine reward system within the brain, thus also causing Parkinson's disease later on in life.

Chagas disease is also a nasty part that can come as a side effect from vagus nerve damage. This disease is known to especially spread itself through the parasympathetic part of the nervous system, and from there it branches off of the vagus nerve, causing destruction as it goes.

When the vagus nerve gets damaged, it is no longer able to send signals through to your digestive system or communicate with the muscles in your stomach, so this may end up causing your food to sit in your digestive system for longer periods of time and ultimately causing you to become severely ill, instead of just moving its way normally through the small intestine in order to be digested.

Certain medications may also lead to a delay in gastric emptying such as painkillers and opioids, certain antidepressants and antianxiety medications, high blood pressure medications, and allergy medications, which can all lead up to some similar symptoms to vagus nerve damage. For those patients who already have gastroparesis, these particular medications may make the condition much worse.

If there are any signs or symptoms that worry you or cause you to think that you may have a damaged vagus nerve, it is best to consult with your nearest doctor or family health practitioner with regards to the symptoms, as they will be able to put your vagus nerve through a number of tests to check whether it may be damaged or not.

There are a number of factors that may increase your risk and chances of getting gastroparesis such as the following:

- Diabetes
- Abdominal or esophageal surgery
- Certain medications that slow the rate of stomach emptying, such as opioids
- Scleroderma of the nerve tissue
- Infection, usually a virus
- Parkinson's disease
- Multiple sclerosis
- Low thyroid

Unfortunately for the lovely ladies of our planet, it has been found that women are more likely to develop gastroparesis than men are.

Gastroparesis can cause several complications, such as:

- Severe dehydration due to vomiting and nausea. If you battle to keep any liquids down you are likely to dehydrate a lot faster.
- Malnutrition due to poor appetite when you aren't taking in enough nutrients in your system or taking in enough calories due to poor appetite.

Vomiting can also lead to a lack of nutrients being absorbed.

- Undigested food which can cause a great deal of harm in the sense that it can harden into a ball in your stomach and not be able to pass through your system. This solid ball of food in your stomach is called a bezoar (it even sounds vicious, doesn't it?) and this delightfully uncomfortable ball can often result in vomiting, and may result in a surgical removal as it can be life threatening to not be able to pass anything through your small intestine past the ball. It is often quite painful too, as it blocks the way for anything further to pass like a foreign body inside your digestive tract.

- Blood sugar changes that can be quite unpredictable. Although gastroparesis isn't directly caused by diabetes, the frequent changes in the rate and amount of food passing into the small bowel can lead to changes in your blood sugar levels that may ultimately lead to diabetes in the future, or cause current diabetes to severely worsen. In turn, a lack of control of blood sugar levels with regards to your diet makes gastroparesis worse.

- Decreased quality of life is a definite. An acute flare-up of painful symptoms may make it tough on you to keep up with your current lifestyle and responsibilities. You may often find yourself sitting there unable to perform common tasks that you have been able to complete with no problems before.

Diabetes can also be a large factor in causing severe nerve damage in its destructive pathway. This can in fact happen to a number of nerves within the body. A prolonged increase in blood sugar that has been associated with diabetes can alter nerve chemistry, and damage the blood vessels that support the nerves, in which case you can often find that intermittent fasting can occasionally be recommended for diabetics to keep a hold on the spikes that they may cause to their blood sugar and insulin. This, of course also needs to be thoroughly monitored through a doctor or family healthcare professional and should never be attempted without letting others know of the game plan.

Chronic alcohol abuse is known to cause damage to nerves, especially when it comes to the vagus nerve, which causes a nasty condition that is called alcoholic neuropathy. When alcohol gets abused at a toxic level on a daily basis, the autonomic nervous system which houses the vagus nerve as its star of the show can become heavily poisoned over time. By no longer drinking alcohol for long periods of time, your vagus nerve will be able to heal itself and reverse the damage that is already done, much like how the liver can regenerate after getting liver damage or having a piece removed through surgery.

Vagus nerve damage can also be a result of upper respiratory viral infections. This will generally happen in less severe cases of damage that were due to coughing, runny nasal passages, and congestion. In patients whose symptoms persisted, they found that they got moderately worse and developing a worsened cough, throat clearing and phlegm in their chests, difficulty speaking, and overall tiredness.

The vagus nerve can also potentially be damaged due to surgery within the stomach or intestines. A procedure called laparoscopic hernia fundoplication, used to treat gastric reflux, has been associated with vagus nerve damage.

There are two types of vagus nerve disorders: those that happen when the nerve is underactive and those when the nerve has been overstimulated.

Some other vagus nerve damage symptoms that we have not yet covered include the likes of muscle cramping in the throat which can prevent a person from being able to speak as well as it would cause a vast amount of pain and discomfort to the person who is battling. A person who is prone to contracting peptic ulcers may unfortunately suffer from vagus nerve dysfunction. You can get peptic ulcers not only in the stomach, but also in the lower esophagus, and the first part of the smaller intestines. The nerve dysfunction increases the acid in the stomach which in turn can cause major cramping and pain. Symptoms of having a peptic ulcer include a burning sensation in the stomach due to the buildup of acid, nausea, and/or vomiting, bloating alongside abdominal pain, and more. Other patients or sufferers of vagus nerve dysfunction may develop constipation issues. The intestines are not regulating the intake of water properly and will not be able to move a stool through the bowel with as much ease as you may want it to. This creates a situation where the stool in your bowels may become too hard to pass and a laxative may be needed. Other people may find that they have an incontinence problem where they no longer have any control over their urinary tract.

Anxiety, depression, fatigue, migraines, memory disorders, bad circulation, arthritis, and so much more can be treated by stimulating the vagus nerve.

Understanding your symptoms is important. It will help your doctor to determine the best course of treatment for you. Stimulating the vagus nerve is the goal. Which route to take in stimulating the vagus nerve is the puzzle.

Treatment for Damage

For some people, they may find that their dysfunction requires electrical stimulation.

This is where the ever so handy vagus nerve stimulator device comes in. It is a special little electronic device that is placed under the skin of your chest or neck and from there it sends signals to the vagus nerve in order to stimulate it. As mentioned, this device is similar to that of a pacemaker for heart patients. This is often one of the first recommended treatments for a vagus nerve with severe damage along the way. You can also try one of the main at home methods that have been previously mentioned during the book and within our passive activities list.

To do a quick recap on where we are so far, we have discussed the vagus nerve location and function in the body. We talked about what can go wrong with the vagus nerve as well as ways to strengthen and treat it. We have discovered that the human body's complexity can make it incredibly difficult to pinpoint the origin of a disease or problem in the system. We have discussed ways in which the vagus nerve can be stimulated to strengthen it after it has been damaged in any way.

You can treat vagus nerve damage at home with care on the basis that it has not reached a life threatening severity. Choosing exactly which method works for your body to maintain your health and a healthy lifestyle is incredibly important in the long run as this is your body that you need to take care of. Gentle exercise can be incredibly good for you and will not harm you in any way as long as it is done properly, especially while your vagus nerve is healing from some sort of trauma. If you give any of our more advanced, yoga- type exercises a try and you are a beginner, try to find a teacher- led class that may be able to give you a hand when you are upside down and looking something like a pretzel. If you are battling with any of these exercises, then a teacher will be able to guide and help you and correct any poses so that you may reap all the benefits in the long run from the exercise. Choosing the correct form of treatment is also something that should be discussed in detail with your medical practitioner.

It would also be a good idea to get somebody trusted, such as a close friend or family member, who could also help you through the challenging times ahead and keep you on track.

Sometimes it's almost easy to say that we can combat this by simply keeping control of our vagus nerve and strengthening it through stimulation or even by seeing a doctor, but a big part of the healing process is also to have a good support system at your back. When you have people who are aware of the problem and are able to give you emotional support along the way, you will be far more likely to stay calm during the process and know that you aren't alone, which will also keep you on the right track when completely giving up starts to look good. Find an emotional partner who can hold you accountable and tackle this problem head-on.

Chapter 6: What Happens With Overstimulation?

The Most Common Cause of Fainting

Why do people drop down in a faint? Something may have frightened them or something may be wrong with their blood pressure perhaps, and they just keel over on the floor without warning. This less than fun little moment that these people have is greatly due to their vagus nerve being under a sudden jolt of stress, pain, or anguish that makes it overreact and the person's brain will momentarily switch off.

When the vagus nerve is busy overreacting, it loses the control that it had over the heart muscles which normally results in a sudden drop in blood pressure and heart rate, resulting in the person either dropping down with no warning, or feeling as though they may be about to faint, giving them enough time to sit on a chair or on the floor so as not to hurt themselves. This is also referred to as vasovagal syncope.

When vasovagal syncope occurs, the person who is unfortunately stuck in its grips will lose consciousness for a few seconds to minutes at time due vastly to the overstimulation of the vagus nerve. But why does this happen? Let us have a look into the steps leading up to the person fainting due to the vagus nerve's overreaction.

The vagus nerve's main role throughout the body (if you could even give it a main role considering how much it does) is to slow down the heart rate of a person when it gets too overexcited. When this signal is given, the vagus nerve ensures that there is less blood being pumped into the arteries which therefore will cause the brain to become less oxygenated as well as drop a person's blood pressure to normal or below instead of being raised to dangerous levels.

Most of the time, when this nerve is overstimulated, it may not present any immediate dangers or complications with a person's body. When it does get to a point of chaos in the body, the body will faint. When these fainting spells are quite lengthy, it is known as syncope.

These are a few of the signs that a person can look out for to identify if they are about to faint before unconsciousness sets in:

- Sudden feeling of weakness will set in, where the body feels like it is almost too heavy to hold up. You may be doing something or carrying an item and find that you have to put it down before you drop it, not because it is heavy, but because your body is unable to take the strain at that moment in time.
- You may also find that you get a sense of vertigo. This is when you lose your balance normally due to an imbalance of fluid in your ears or caused by

an ear infection. The world will spin around you a bit during this time.

- Blurry vision is your next sign that you might be about to faint. This can often present itself like waves in your vision, or some people have described it as looking like TV fuzz when your bunny-ear aerial isn't playing along. If you can wrap your head around this one, you could almost say that your vision looks a bit like how sparkling water tastes. Bubbly!

- Hot flashes can also be problematic in this department. You may feel like your face goes completely hot, like someone is holding a match up to your forehead. This can also sometimes be paired with the symptom of going red and flushed. This is all due to the blood rushing to your brain in an 'emergency' case of going straight to the vital organs when the pressure is low.

- Sweating is also going to accompany these hot flashes. There unfortunately is no way of avoiding it, but you will most likely break out into a sweat whether you are hot in the sun or sitting in an airconditioned room when you're feeling faint.

- Last but not least you may find a nasty ringing in your ears. Some people have also described that when somebody had been talking to them, it may have sounded like they were under water or that their ears were horribly blocked.

Since the vagus nerve also plays such a large role in the digestive system, you may also find that a person experiences a level of nausea and vomiting before or after a fainting spell.

The vagus nerve may even surprise you further and cause diarrhea after a fainting spell as the digestive system becomes completely relaxed and is unable to hold anything in, nor will it be able to allow the intestines to get any nutrients or water out of your food.

While going through a fainting spell can be a major symptom of your vagus nerve overreacting in the short term, vagus nerve dysfunction can also have a number of long term symptoms that can show up during your lifetime. The symptoms include Irritable Bowel Syndrome, sudden weight loss or weight gain than can become quite extreme over time, excessive anxiety, as well as chronic fatigue that is crippling. If you do find that these symptoms are affecting you along with your vagus nerve dysfunction, you can speak to your doctor or healthcare practitioner to see if there is a treatment best suited to relieve these particular symptoms.

There are a number of factors surrounding vagus nerve dysfunction that we have found to be high contributors. Certain medications, for example, can trigger vagus nerve dysfunction, especially heart medications and those in use for high or low blood pressure. Another major contributing factor is a person's mental and psychological state of mind.

Circumstances that put people into high levels of stress or give off a strong surge of emotion, such as seeing blood when a person has a phobia, can wreak havoc on how a dysfunctional vagus nerve works. Physical problems that can cause a person to feel uncomfortable may also play a role here, such as an overly hot and uncomfortable atmosphere, prolonged standing in one spot (which includes the pain of standing during pregnancy), pregnancy itself in general, especially during the last trimester when everything requires that much more effort, as well as intense physical pain can each in their own way stimulate the vagus nerve and act as a trigger towards vagus nerve dysfunction.

What do you do in a case where you are experiencing vagus nerve dysfunction? Should this happen to you and any of the signs or symptoms are staring you in the face, your best option according to first aid is to lie down and raise your legs so that they are above your heart.

Hold this spot for a few minutes in order to allow the blood in your system to move more freely to your heart and brain when your pressure is low and the vital organs need it most to keep you conscious. By raising your legs, you are able to restore your body's normal blood pressure. If you are not sure if you are experiencing some level of vagus nerve dysfunction or not, it is advised to ask somebody for help as soon as possible, as in some cases should you suddenly lose consciousness, you may fall or experience some form of trauma.

Finding the Perfect Balance

Sometimes, and maybe more often than we actually care to admit to ourselves, the easily accessible power that the vagus nerve holds in order to reduce inflammation and anxiety gets underestimated and overlooked as a method of balanced treatment for the body.

We are often far too quick to reach for Ibuprofen and Prozac, and don't always realize that we have to tools to balance our lives right in the palm of...well, not our hands specifically, but in our nervous system and waiting to be used.

You could almost go as far as to say that the vagus nerve has its own type of 'yin yang' factor to it.

By this I mean that with the vagus nerve we have both the sympathetic and parasympathetic nervous systems that are polar opposites in what they do. On the sympathetic side, you have you fight or flight mode that gives you a burst of adrenaline and cortisol in order to pounce on whatever may be about to attack you (currently in my case, a spider that is eyeballing me from the wall opposite where I am sitting), while on the other hand, your parasympathetic nerve which allows you to relax and lower your breathing and heart rate after the burst of energy previously felt. (I think I will name him Michael). So when Michael decides to shimmey his way back out the window to his little spider family, my parasympathetic nervous system can kick in and allow me to breathe again!

The tug of war in a push and pull fight between these two sides of the nervous system thus creates the ultimate balance within your body with homeostasis.

If we go back in time, and I mean many, many years, we could look at the possibilities from an evolutionary perspective, too. We could probably say that our ancestors relied on the sympathetic nervous system in order to get their instincts for hunting as well as to stay safe against any enemies that could potentially attack them or steal their food supply.

On the other hand, the parasympathetic nervous system probably allowed others in the family tree to bond between and make sure that the family was cared for as well as to ensure procreation of the next generation and build supportive communities amongst themselves.

Sadly for the rest of us, the 21st century has caused a lot of change over a short period of time that we, as the next generation, have had to struggle to keep up with the times.

This in turn is causing our systems to completely short circuit more often than not, and we are having to go all out to keep the balance necessary for our body's survival. Our nervous systems have no idea what is going on these days! Recent studies have shown that social media and other modern-day technological factors are causing far more social isolation, anxiety, depression, and feelings of being unworthy of love. On top of that, we have made it a habit to have "every man for himself" becoming the norm which can also throw off some people's fight and flight responses, as you don't have anyone that you can turn to should you need physical or emotional help.

Fortunately, the last few generations have figured out how we can use the vagus nerve to our benefit, and this is slowly developing its way into a full rolling therapy treatment for many people. Researchers are still to this day and minute finding new ways to use the vagus nerve to our advantage, and tweaking it in just the right way to get the full power.

What is marvelous about this life balancing technique of vagus nerve stimulation is that it doesn't have to cost you a cent. With most cases being something that you can stimulate your nerve with at home and only a few that require a vagus nerve stimulator, it can put the power into your own hands and allow for a better quality of life overall.

Interesting Facts About the Vagus Nerve

- The vagus nerve comes from a Latin name "Vaga", and is considered to be a wandering nerve much like a vagabond would wander, thus some may call it the vagabond nerve. It is also known as the "wandering nerve" because it has multiple branches that diverge from two thick stems rooted in the cerebellum and brainstem that wander to the lowest viscera of your abdomen, touching your heart and most major organs along the way.
- The vagus nerve is fantastic for preventing inflammation. Having a small amount of inflammation during illness is quite alright, but when it gets out of hand it is often then linked with

a number of conditions such as arthritis. When the vagus nerve gets a signal to say that there is inflammation in the body due to there being cytokines present in the body, the vagus nerve will then respond quickly to the brain in order to activate its anti-inflammatory neurotransmitters in order to allow the body's immune system to regulate.

- The vagus nerve is also incredibly well-known for helping your brain to develop memories! Studies were done with rats in a University in Virginia that showed that stimulating the vagus nerves of these rats had greatly strengthened their memories. This is due to a neurotransmitter called norepinephrine, which gets released into the amygdala of the brain where memories are formed and thrive. Other studies that had been done on humans had also found incredible results with regards to a future treatment for conditions such as Alzheimer's disease as well as dementia.

- The vagus nerve is also known to assist with the body's need to breathe. A neurotransmitter called acetylcholine that is created by the vagus nerve is what gets triggered in order to let your lungs know that now is a good time to inhale and exhale for the sake of survival. Did you know that this is also why the use of Botox in any cosmetic types of surgeries can be potentially dangerous to your overall health? This is because the use of Botox is known to mess with the production of the acetylcholine neurotransmitter which in turn would prevent you from being able to breathe. On the bright side though, this is where the power gets put in your own hands with stimulating breathing exercises that can help you to strengthen your vagus nerve by yourself.

- The neurotransmitter called acetylcholine was the first-ever neurotransmitter discovered by scientists and got its name originally from a physiologist named Otto Leowi, who learnt of the substance through causing a reduction in heart rate during a vagus nerve study. He called the substance 'Vagusstoff' which is directly translated from German for "vagus substance".
- Much like how the vagus nerve is very intimately related to your lungs, it is equally related to your heart. Using specific electrical impulses through to the heart muscles, the vagus nerve can control your heart rate somewhat like a pacemaker. Doctors will generally use this information by measuring your heart rate variability between your individual heart beats over time in order to know whether anything may be wrong with your ticker. To do this they work very closely with the vagus nerve.
- The vagus nerve is completely responsible for keeping up with your body's relaxation response. As the vagus nerve is the part of your body that creates the neurotransmitter acetylcholine, it is what is responsible for getting your body to calm down when your sympathetic nervous system has a 'freak out' moment and releases adrenaline and

cortisol into your blood. By having the tendrils of the vagus nerve connected to each of your vital organs, your body is able to release the proteins and enzymes needed to relax you such as prolactin, oxytocin, and vasopressin.

- A person is more likely to have a speedy recovery from illness, injury, or stress when they have a strengthened vagus nerve. They are able to strengthen their vagus nerve through any of the techniques that we have mentioned in this book.

- Your vagus nerve acts as a walkie-talkie between your digestive system and your brain. Electrical impulses are sent between your gut and your brain to tell you whether you may be feeling nauseous, sore, or even to tell you that something is making you nervous or anxious. You shouldn't ignore your "gut feelings." They are often right and know what is best for you and your body!

- Just as we discussed earlier, fun fact: overstimulation of your vagus nerve is by far the most common cause of a person fainting. If you are feeling faint because of a fear such as the fear of needles or blood, it isn't because you're a baby or weak, but because your vagus nerve has been overstimulated in a short span of time and you are now getting what is called 'vagal syncope.' Your body responds to the sudden stress by quite literally turning itself off like a lightswitch as the blood in your brain is restricted and you ultimately end up losing consciousness. By lying down or sitting and breathing, you may be able to alleviate the symptoms before you drop.

- The vagus nerve has been known to greatly reduce the signs of inflammation through electronic stimulation. Studies were done on rats in order to determine whether stimulation of the vagus nerve would be able to reduce inflammation in the rat and the results were so successful that the study was moved onto humans with exceptional results, showing that it may inhibit the inflammation altogether. By using a vagus nerve stimulating implant that allowed for the vagus nerve to be stimulated electronically, a drastic reduction in inflammation was shown as well as remission on arthritis which has no true known cure and is often only treated with anti-inflammatory medications.
- Scientists and doctors are currently working on replacing medications and high schedule drugs with vagus nerve stimulation devices. Since vagal nerve stimulation has shown such high success in the treatment of epilepsy, inflammation, and depression, a new medical field known as bioelectric has come into play as the future of medicine as we know it. With these new studies, scientists and doctors are hoping to be able to treat illness and injury with as few side effects as possible in the long run.

Conclusion

Now that you have been armed with the world's greatest secrets to unlocking your body's new potential, what will you do with them? It is now time to start your healing process, no matter what ailment you may be experiencing. Use the power of the vagus nerve to unlock your beauty and power within, reduce your stress levels, and find the ultimate level of calm within yourself! Life just unlocked a whole new world of opportunity.

References

Crumrine, P-Vagal Nerve Stimulation in Children retrieved from: https://www.ncbi.nlm.nih.gov/pubmed/11023179

Delgado, J- Vagus Nerve and Anxiety: Everything You Need To Know retrieved from: https://psychology-spot.com/vagus-nerve-anxiety/

Fogoros, R (2019). The Role Of the Vagus Nerve in the Nervous System retrieved from: https://www.verywellhealth.com/vagus-nerve-anatomy-174612

McIntyre, C (2018). Is There a Role For Vagus Nerve Stimulation in the Treatment Of Posttraumatic Stress Disorder? retrieved from: https://www.futuremedicine.com/doi/10.2217/bem-2018-0002

Parnell, G (2018). How To Treat Vagus Nerve Damage At Home retrieved from: https://nerve-injury.com/vagus-nerve-damage

Richardson, MW (2019). Are Commercial Vagus Nerve Stimulation Devices Safe and Effective? retrieved from: https://www.brainfacts.org/diseases-and-disorders/therapies/2019/are-commercial-vagus-nerve-stimulation-devices-safe-and-effective-042419

Ropp, T (2017). 12 Ways To Unlock the Powers Of the Vagus Nerve retrieved from: https://upliftconnect.com/12-ways-unlock-powers-vagus-nerve/

Rosenfeld, J (2018). 9 Fascinating Facts About the Vagus Nerve retrieved from: http://mentalfloss.com/article/65710/9-nervy-facts-about-vagus-nerve

Schwartz, A (2019). The Vagus Nerve in Trauma Recovery: retrieved from: https://drarielleschwartz.com/the-vagus-nerve-in-trauma-recovery-dr-arielle-schwartz/#.XaHT0ZIzbIU

Seymour,T (2017). Vagus Nerve. Function, Stimulation, and Further Research retrieved from: https://www.medicalnewstoday.com/articles/318128.php

Weinberg, J (2018). Reducing Inflammation Starts with the Vagus Nerve retrieved from: https://chopra.com/articles/reducing-inflammation-starts-with-the-vagus-nerve

Wikipedia - Vagus Nerve retrieved from: https://en.wikipedia.org/wiki/Vagus_nerve

CPSIA information can be obtained
at www.ICGtesting.com
Printed in the USA
BVHW042108100222
628699BV00012B/403

9 781801 119696